*"Addiction, like the ocean,
is immeasurable by the surface."*

The Addiction/Trauma Workbook

*Guide Your
Personal Recovery*

Lori Marmoreo, MSN

A donation of the workbook proceeds will be given to individuals beginning residential treatment for substance dependency/addiction.

I have partnered with my dear friend, Jessica Dawson, who has already begun to help people in need, through her non-profit organization (SAW).

About the Author

Lori Marmoreo, MSN, is a Masters prepared retired Registered Nurse of 33 years and a University Professor. She is also holds a Certificate in Addiction Treatment and Care (UBC).

Lori is a recovering addict/alcoholic, which makes this workbook unique.

Lori has combined her professional knowledge with her personal experience in the creation of her workbook, in order to help you build a comprehensive recovery plan based on your own life experiences.

Overall, this undertaking has brought Lori to a new state of peace.

She hopes the same happens for you.

Lori has left no stone unturned in attempt to help you understand and manage *your* substance dependency. While this workbook cannot guarantee recovery, it will provide *you* with a *tailored framework* of your personal experiences in order to devise a plan of recovery specifically designed for *you*, by *you*. This workbook may be an excellent accessory for *you* and *your recovery team* to work with.

Dedication

To my father Charles and step-mother Bonnie; My children- Chris, Carley, & Hannah; my husband John; and my sister Lynda, for not giving up on me. You knew that I wasn't strong enough to pull my self out; that's when you all stepped in. Thank you for saving my life.

To the exceptional staff at Freedom From Addiction Rehabilitation Center, with special recognition to Jay Albi, Lisa Herron, and Liz Bloom for their expertise and compassion.

To our dear brother, Cheech. The world lost a really great man the day you went to heaven. You made a great impact in my recovery and a bigger impact in the hearts of many, especially Allie and me. You made us feel alive and happy when we had forgotten what that felt like. The energy changed when you entered a room and your encouragement made us feel like we could handle anything—you were a positive bright light, and for that, you will live on in our hearts forever. We know you are looking down on us and cheering us on, as we continue on our journey of life because we all know addiction is a beast and too many of us don't make it out alive. Until we meet again brother, rest peacefully. Love mama bear.

Finally, I dedicate this workbook to those who currently suffer in active addiction, and to you!

You've made it this far. Please don't give up on yourself.

GENERAL DISCLAIMER:

The use of "The Addiction Workbook" implies your acceptance of this disclaimer:

This publication is a diverse source of inspirational information.

The ideas, suggestions, and questionnaires contained in this book are not intended to replace the services of trained professionals, nor was it designed to provide medical advice.

Any person or entity reading this publication agrees to release and discharge the author and publisher, from any and all claims of liability, obligation, or responsibility, expressed or implied; or adverse effects, alleged to have happened directly or indirectly as a consequence from the information contained in this book.

If you have or suspect you may have a health problem, consult your health care provider.

If you believe you have a medical emergency, call 911 immediately.

Copyrighted Material
The Addiction/Trauma Workbook
Copyright © 2022 by Lori Marmoreo. All Rights Reserved.

No part of this publication may be reproduced, stored in a retrieval system or transmitted, in any form or by any means—electronic, mechanical, photocopy, recording, or otherwise—without prior written permission from the publisher, except for the inclusion of brief quotations in a review.

For information about this title or to order other books and/or electronic media, contact the publisher:

Lori Marmoreo
email: TheATWorkbook@gmail.com

ISBN: 978-1-7780458-0-6 (paperback)
ISBN: 978-1-7780458-1-3 (ebook)

Printed in the United States of America

Book & cover design: www.van-garde.com
Cover photo: LaLima Design

Contents

1. Introduction 1
2. Medical Addiction Questionnaires 3
    DSM-IV Questionnaire: 3
    DAST-10 Questionnaire: 5
3. Johns Hopkins University Hospital Addiction Questionnaire 8
4. The Diagnostic Criteria for Alcohol Withdrawal
   Syndrome Questionnaire (DSM-5) 11
5. Clinical Opiate Withdrawal Scale (COWS) Questionnaire 13
6. Addiction Behaviors/Personality Characteristics 15
7. Biology of the Brain 17
    World Health Organization, WHO: 17
    Healing the Brain (Yale University Research) 18
8. The Trauma Informed Practice Guide 19
9. Abuse 23
10. Anxiety 32
11. Depression 36
12. General Questions 42
13. The Stages of Change 68
14. Powerlessness and Unmanageability 70
15. Ambivalence 73
16. Dangerous Thought Pathway 76
17. Triggers 77
18. Shame and Guilt 79
19. Regret 84
20. Inner Critic 86
21. Psychology Tools/Unhelpful Thinking Styles 88
22. Inner Child 92

23.	Boundaries	97
24.	Trust	101
25.	Personal Values	104
26.	Love/Relationships	110
27.	Play	115
28.	Friendships	118
29.	Purpose and Spirituality	122
30.	Gratitude	124
31.	Anger	127
32.	Anger Assignment	137
33.	Resentment	140
34.	Fear	144
35.	The 7 Stages of Grief	145
36.	Post Acute Withdrawal	149
37.	SMART Framework	152
38.	Goal-Setting Strategies	157
39.	Maslow's Hierarchy of Needs	159
40.	Alternative Therapies	162
	Cognitive Behavioral Therapy (CBT)	162
	Mindfulness	162
	Self-care	162
	Reiki	162
	Meditation	163
	Balance	164
41.	Connectedness	166
42.	Honesty	167
43.	Morals	169
44.	Symptoms of Stress	171
45.	Myths About Recovery	173

46. Daily Inventory/Recovery Checklists 174
47. Relapse Behaviors & Treatment 177
48. Relapse Symptoms/Emergency Tool Kit 179
49. The Addiction Crisis and Government Responsibilities 184
50. Alcohol 188
    The History of Alcohol 188
    The Temperance Movement 188
    Effects of Alcohol on Society 189
51. Conclusion 190
52. I Am Your Disease 193
53 Your Personal Summary Page(s) 196
54. Your Health & Personal Recovery Plan 248
55. My Story 263
56. References 271

1. Introduction

> *"You put up walls so high that only the crazy would climb them to be with you…well, here I am!"*

My intention with this workbook is simple – at optimum, it may: shift *your* perspective, lighten *your* burden, and increase *your* knowledge of *your* addiction. It was designed for *you* to answer questions about *your* life experiences in order for *you* to understand how addiction has affected *your* life.

This is not a competition or a race; there is no time limit or exam at the end. Do this at your own pace, but do it!

You will begin to understand yourself on a new level, which will boost your personal growth.

> *"ONE DAY or DAY ONE, you decide."*

What will you lose by staying sober versus if you don't? Wouldn't it be easier to go through life accepting you have an addiction, rather that trying to convince everyone else that you don't?

Well, the good news is that you are reading this right now; you are willing to fight for your life and I can help you begin the process.

It's time to get out of survival mode. New habits = New life, because when you carry the bricks from your past, you will build the same house.

> *"It is not the strongest of the species that survives, nor the most intelligent—it is the one that is most adaptable to change."*
> —Charles Darwin

What are you waiting for?

START NOW.
START WHERE YOU ARE.
START WITH YOUR MIND RACING.
START WITH YOUR HANDS SHAKING.
START WITH DOUBT.
START WITH FEAR, BUT START.
JUST START!

Only a licensed medical professional is able to diagnose whether or not you have a substance dependency. This workbook may simply give you an idea of where you're at today. Refer to the disclaimer at the beginning of this book for important information before you proceed.

Additionally, I feel it is important for you to know a bit about who is helping you and the experiences I have also faced, therefore my story of addiction and trauma are included in "My Story" at the end of the workbook.

"Addiction is not a badness; it's a disease."

The scrutiny of addiction is that it is a moral choice, which is a malicious and prevalent view. In reality, it's far different.

The American College of Physicians classifies alcoholism as a disease (American Psychiatric Association, 1994).

There is not one medical professional organization that does not agree, "addiction is a chronic illness, and although it can be successfully treated, it cannot be cured" (Adlersberg 1997; Chychula & Sciamanna, 2002; Maddux & Desmond, 2000).

What tool do medical professionals use to diagnose addiction/substance dependency?

2. Medical Addiction Questionnaires

One of the tools medical professionals use to diagnose substance dependency, or addiction, is *the Diagnostic and Statistical Manual of Mental Disorders (DSM-IV);* asks a series of questions to determine if you may have an issue with addiction, or substance dependency (American Psychiatric Association, 2013).

(If your "addiction" is something other than alcohol, then substitute it for the word *alcohol* below).

DSM-IV Questionnaire:
Have any of the following occurred at any time in the same 12-month period?

Please circle Y=yes or N=no for the following questions:

1. Substance is often taken in larger amounts or over a longer period than was intended   Y/N

2. There is persistent desire or unsuccessful efforts to cut down or control substance use   Y/N

3. A great deal of time is spent in activities necessary to obtain substance, or recover from its effects   Y/N

4. Craving or a strong desire or urge to use substance   Y/N

5. Recurrent substance use has resulted in a failure to fulfill major role obligations at work, school, or home   Y/N

6. Continued substance use despite having persistent or recurrent social or interpersonal problems caused or exacerbated by the effects of substance   Y/N

7. Important social, occupational, or recreational activities are given up or reduced because of substance use   Y/N

8. Recurrent substance use in situations in which it is physically hazardous   Y/N

9. Continued use despite knowledge of having persistent or recurrent physical or psychological problems that is likely to have been caused or exacerbated by the substance   Y/N

10. Tolerance, as defined by either of the following

    a. A need for markedly increased amounts of the substance to achieve intoxication or the desired effect

    b. A markedly diminished effect with continued use of the same substance   Y/N

11. Withdrawal, as manifested by either of the following:

    a. The characteristic withdrawal for the substance

    b. The same (or closely related) substance is taken to relieve or avoid withdrawal symptoms   Y/N

(Note: This criterion is not considered met for those taking prescription opiates solely under medical supervision).

Severity: Mild: 2–3 symptoms, Moderate: 4–5 symptoms, Severe: 6 or more symptoms.

How many did you answer "yes" to___/11?

If you answered yes to 2 or more of the questions above, you have substance use disorder.

In early remission: 3 months clean/sober but for less that 12 months (with exception of #4).

In sustained remission: 12 months or longer

Transfer your score and comments onto your personal summary page.

DAST-10 Questionnaire:

The *Drug Abuse Screening Test (DAST-10)*, is another diagnostic tool used by medical professionals to diagnose drug addiction: (The Addiction Research Foundation, 1982).

The following are a list of questions concerning what your potential involvement is with drugs, excluding alcohol and tobacco, during the past 12 months.

When the terms "drug abuse" are mentioned in the questions below, they mean taken in excess of the directions and any non-medical use of drugs e.g., cannabis (marijuana, hash); solvents; tranquilizers (e.g. Valium); barbiturates, cocaine, stimulants (e.g., speed); hallucinogens, (e.g. LSD), or narcotics (e.g. heroin). Remember the questions do not include alcohol or tobacco.

If you have difficulty with a statement, then choose what is mostly right.

These questions refer to the past 12 months:

1. Have you used drugs other than those required for medical reasons?   Y/N

2. Do you abuse more than one drug at a time?   Y/N

3. Are you always able to stop using drugs when you want to? If you never use drugs, answer "Yes"   Y/N

4. Have you had "blackouts" or "flashbacks" as a result of drug use?   Y/N

5. Do you ever feel bad or guilty about your drug use? If never use drugs, choose "No"   Y/N

6. Does your spouse (or parents) ever complain about your involvement with drugs?   Y/N

7. Have you neglected your family because of your use of drugs?   Y/N

8. Have you engaged in illegal activities in order to obtain drugs?   Y/N

9. Have you ever experienced withdrawal symptoms (felt sick) when you stopped taking drugs?   Y/N

10. Have you had medical problems as a result of your drug use? (e.g., memory loss, hepatitis, convulsions, bleeding, etc.)   Y/N

How many did you answer "yes" to____/10?

How many did you answer "no" to ____/10?

Interpreting the DAST-10:

In these statements, the term "drug use" refers to the use of medications at a level that exceeds the instructions, and/or any non-medical use of drugs.

Patients receive 1-point for every "yes" answer with the exception of question #3, for which a "no" answer receives 1-point. DAST-10 Score Degree of Problems Related to Drug Abuse Suggested Action:

DAST-10 Score	Degree of Problems Related to Drug Abuse	Suggested Action
0	No problems reported	None at this time
1–2	Low level	Monitor, re-assess at a later date
3–5	Moderate level	Further investigation

6–8	Substantial level	Intensive assessment
9–10	Severe level	Intensive assessment

Transfer your score and comments onto your personal summary page.

How did answering those questions make you feel?

Something to keep in mind:

> "People who do not have an addiction to alcohol don't have to promise not to drink; they don't have to have to limit themselves; or have to change what they drink so they don't get as inebriated."

3. Johns Hopkins University Hospital Addiction Questionnaire

Let's do another questionnaire.

20—Question Addiction Questionnaire John Hopkins (http://www.badgeoflifecanada.org).

John Hopkins University Hospital in Baltimore, Maryland, developed the following *self—test* for alcoholism and addiction:

(If you're addicted to something other than drugs, substitute for *use/using* below).

1. Do you lose time from work due to using?   Y/N

2. Is using making your home life unhappy?   Y/N

3. Do you use because you are shy with other people?   Y/N

4. Is using affecting your reputation?   Y/N

5. Have you ever felt remorse after using?   Y/N

6. Have you gotten into financial difficulties as a result of using?   Y/N

7. Do you turn to companions or go to an area you normally wouldn't if you weren't using or seeking your drug?   Y/N

8. Does your use make you careless of your family's welfare?   Y/N

9. Has your ambition decreased since you started using?   Y/N

10. Do you have cravings at a definite time daily?   Y/N

11. Do you want to use the next morning?   Y/N

12. Does using cause you to have difficulty with sleeping?   Y/N

13. Has your efficiency decreased since you began using?   Y/N

14. Is using jeopardizing your job or business?   Y/N

15. Do you use to escape worries, stress, or trouble?   Y/N

16. Do you use alone?   Y/N

17. Have you ever had a complete loss of memory as a result of using?   Y/N

18. Has your doctor ever treated you for this?   Y/N

19. Do you use to build up your self-confidence?   Y/N

20. Have you ever been to a hospital or institution on account of using?   Y/N

How many did you answer "yes" to____/20?

If you have answered "yes" to 3 questions, it suggests you probably have a drinking or drug problem.

If you have answered "yes" to 4–7 questions, it suggests you may be in an early stage of alcoholism or drug addiction.

If you have answered "yes" to 7–10 questions, it suggests you may be in the second stage of alcoholism or drug addiction.

If you answered "yes" to more than 10 questions, it suggests you may be in end-stage alcoholism or drug addiction.

Transfer your score and comments onto your personal summary page.

How do you feel right now? Are you ok? Take a short break if you need to.

Ask yourself, did you try to deny any of your answers or try to keep your "yes" answers to fewer than two? I did, but the only person I was trying to convince was myself! I felt way too vulnerable answering truthfully—because, then, I couldn't hide. I wasn't ready.

When I tried to soften my answers, I relapsed twice. The third time I relapsed, I totally surrendered and finally answered all of the questions truthfully. I had to push myself to do this because even though I knew that I needed to,

I was still afraid. I was fearful that somebody would read my answers and use them against me. So, I understand how you are feeling. Just remember, freedom is on the other side of fear.

When I answered the 20 questions truthfully, I got 20/20. It was a double-edged sword. I knew I was at rock bottom, but seeing this was a wake-up call. I was sick of being in active addiction and I was ready to get help.

"Perfect alibis are no longer required."

4. The Diagnostic Criteria for Alcohol Withdrawal Syndrome Questionnaire (DSM-5)

The next 2 medical questionnaires address alcohol withdrawal and opiate withdrawal (drugs).

Ready? Lets do an Alcohol withdrawal questionnaire.

DSM-IV Diagnostic Criteria for Alcohol Withdrawal Syndrome (American Psychiatric Association, 1994):

    A.   Cessation of (or reduction in) alcohol use that has been heavy and prolonged   Y/N

    B.   Two (or more) of the following, developing within several hours to a few days after the cessation of (or reduction in) alcohol use described in Criterion A:

- Autonomic hyperactivity (e.g., sweating or pulse rate greater than 100 beats per minute)   Y/N
- Increased hand tremor   Y/N
- Insomnia   Y/N
- Nausea or vomiting   Y/N
- Transient visual, tactile, or auditory hallucinations or illusions   Y/N
- Psychomotor agitation   Y/N
- Anxiety   Y/N

How many did you answer "yes" to ___/8?

For most people alcohol withdrawal symptoms are mild to moderate and resolve quickly.

Symptoms of alcohol withdrawal typically begin 6–24 hours after the last drink, and reach peak intensity at 24–72 hours, and improve within 7 days" (Alcohol Withdrawal Syndrome - Wikipedia, 2022).

Transfer your score and comments onto your personal summary page.

What are opiates?

Examples of opiates are Oxycodone ("Percs" Percocet), Hydrocodone, Hydromorphone ("Juice" Dilaudid), ("M" Morphine), Fentanyl, Codeine (Tylenol 1's, 2's, 3',s 4's), ("Meth" Methadone), Demerol, Tramadol, Buprenorphine and Carfentanil (Prescription Opioids/CAMH, 2022).

Opiates are highly addictive, even when prescribed by a physician.

Are you curious to know if you have had opiate withdrawal symptoms? Let's look at a questionnaire about opiate withdrawal.

5. Clinical Opiate Withdrawal Scale (COWS) Questionnaire

The Clinical Opiate Withdrawal Scale, also known as COWS (Wesson, 2003):

1. Resting heart rate greater than 100 beats per minute   Y/N
2. Sweating over past 30 minutes not accounted for by room temperature or physical activity   Y/N
3. Restlessness or feeling unable to sit still   Y/N
4. Pupil size dilated (large)   Y/N
5. Bone or joint aches   Y/N
6. Upset stomach (cramps; nausea; vomiting; diarrhea)   Y/N
7. Tremor, either felt or seen, from mild to twitching   Y/N
8. Yawning (once or more during the assessment)   Y/N
9. Anxieties or Irritability   Y/N
10. Gooseflesh skin (piloerrection of skin-bumps or hairs standing up on arms)   Y/N

How many did you answer "yes" to___/10?

Transfer your score and comments onto your personal summary page.

> *"Cemeteries are full of people who thought they would just use one more time."*

Based on these withdrawal symptoms, we can understand why it is so difficult to quit and not just use one more time.

The problem is that you need more and more opiates in order to get the same effect and this increases your chances of overdosing.

Naloxone (Narcan) is a medication that can temporarily reverse the effects of an opioid overdose (Prescription Opioids/CAMH, 2022). Make no mistake, Naloxone does not reverse the effects of *all* drugs, nor is it a guarantee of survival from opiate overdose.

There is no singular way to stay clean and sober. Your situation is unique. Having said that, one thing you will need to identify the traumatic events that you have been through. Once you identify them, you can begin to work through them. It's vital to take this first step, even if you don't see the whole staircase.

> *"The characteristics of our personality change right before we use, when we use, and after we use."*

6. Addiction Behaviors/Personality Characteristics

The following is a partial list of behaviors exhibited by a person suffering from addiction (gathered from several internet sites, not an exhaustive list): Which ones can you identify with?

1. Controlled or uncontrolled using   Y/N
2. Constant fixation on drug of choice   Y/N
3. Have health problems due to addiction   Y/N
4. Have mood swings (e.g. restless, irritable, aggressive) due to having a low frustration tolerance   Y/N
5. Being preoccupied   Y/N
6. Financial struggles   Y/N
7. Lack motivation and priorities   Y/N
8. Have resentments   Y/N
9. Be dishonest   Y/N
10. Isolate and withdraw from loved ones   Y/N
11. Appear chronically depressed or apathetic   Y/N
12. Personal hygiene is an issue   Y/N
13. Steal from family, friends, and/or strangers   Y/N
14. Promiscuous/risky sexual behavior   Y/N
15. Exhibit strong primitive defense mechanisms such as denial, rationalization, minimization, projection, justifying, blaming   Y/N
16. Relationship issues   Y/N

17. Have difficulty with interpersonal relationships or keeping a job   Y/N

18. Engage in illegal and/or immoral activities to obtain your drug   Y/N

How many did you answer "yes" to___/18?

Rank these troublesome behaviors from 1-18, with 1 being the worse and 18 being the least.

Transfer your score and comments onto your personal summary page.

A drinking story:

When I was on a vacation, I went to an open 12-step meeting where a man told his story about his alcohol addiction.

To my best recollection, he said he had to lie to his wife all the time to say that he wasn't drinking, when he was. He blamed his drinking on loosing his job, and then realized that blaming something or someone was his excuse to drink. His wife felt sorry for him for a while, until his drunkenness became unbearable. He said he had to get really creative in order to hide his alcohol or she'd find it and pour it out! So, guess where he hid his alcohol? Are you ready for this? He replaced his windshield wiper fluid in his car with whiskey!! The vintage car was never driven and stayed in the garage! He laughed and said, "she'd never look in there!" I'm happy to say that he has been sober for over 20 years! He is grateful for his sobriety and now he speaks at 12-step meetings to help others.

Even though he and I have very different stories, we share the commonality of alcohol addiction. I used to hide my bottles in my bedroom drawer, between sweaters, in an old golf bag – wherever I thought they would be concealed.

Please take a short break if you feel overwhelmed.

> *"Strength does not come from physical capacity.*
> *It comes from an indomitable will!"*

7. Biology of the Brain

Now let's review the science of the brain and how it functions in order to have a better understanding of how addiction changes that.

Like our heart, our brain is an organ and operates based on signals or input throughout the body. Everything communicates to deliver the intended message. Transformations in these signals occur from trauma in the prefrontal cortex where we process thoughts and feelings. Specific damage includes defective moral and social reasoning, decision making, and judgment; changes in mood; memory loss; confusion; entropy (lack of order or predictability); loss of empathic reasoning; lowering of the pleasure threshold; and decreasing impulse control, just to name a few.

Our neuro-signals are rerouted to an area in the brain that's not equipped to process them.

The brain's reward system is stimulated by the neurotransmitter dopamine. The hope is that if you can decrease dopamine, which regulates emotions and carries the pleasurable signal, you can loosen the drug's hold on you (Griffith, 1999). When the brain loves something, it craves it, which is why you can't control addiction with willpower alone.

There is a significant correlation between mental health and drug abuse. Removing a substance is only the tip of the iceberg; healing needs to begin in the brain (Griffith, 1999). When the prefrontal cortex gets rerouted, how does it heal?

World Health Organization, WHO:

In 2004, the World Health Organization (WHO) published a detailed report on alcohol and other psychoactive substances, *Neuroscience of psychoactive use and dependence*. This was the first attempt by the WHO to give an overview of the biological factors associated with drug use and dependence, by summarizing the vast amount of information gained over the last 20-30 years. The report states "dependence has not previously been recognized as a brain disorder in the same way that psychiatric and mental illness were not previously recognized as a result of a disorder of the brain, however with recent advances in neuroscience, it is clear that dependence is just as much of a disorder of the brain as any other neurological or psychiatric illness." (WHO, 2004)

Additionally, addiction obliterates focus and discipline. Our conscious mind is responsible for things like morality, judgment, understanding consequences, and loving. When the pleasure center is activated in our subconscious mind, craving is an involuntary response. Thankfully, things such as hope and gratitude stimulate our brain to release healing hormones.

Healing the Brain (Yale University Research)

Researchers at Yale University have reported that 90 days of continuous abstinence begins to restore the decision-making process and analytical functions in the prefrontal cortex! 90 days is a recommended time to be in an inpatient drug-treatment program, not 30. Scientists say extinguishing the cravings is not a matter of eliminating emotions but of helping the addict learn a new kind of conditioning, which allows the midbrain to shut down certain other areas of the brain (Griffith, 1999). Brain damage, from addiction, is actually seen in MRI scans and PET scans. It's real. Thank goodness, it can be "rewired." This information restored my hope that I didn't do irreversible damage to myself.

8. The Trauma Informed Practice Guide

Let's discuss the effects of trauma according to the British Columbia Centre of Excellence for Women's Health: (Understanding Trauma, 2014).

The definitions of trauma from the Trauma Informed Practice Guide are as follows, in order for you to identify with trauma, or not:

1. Single-incident trauma is related to an unexpected and overwhelming event such as an accident, natural disaster, single episode of abuse or assault, sudden loss, or witnessing violence.

2. Complex or repetitive trauma is related to ongoing abuse, domestic violence, war, or ongoing betrayal, often involving being trapped emotionally and/or physically.

3. Developmental trauma results from exposure to early ongoing or repetitive trauma (as infants, children, and youth) involving neglect, abandonment, physical abuse or assault, sexual abuse or assault, emotional abuse, witnessing violence or death, and/or coercion or betrayal. This often occurs within the child's caregiving system and interferes with healthy attachment and development.

4. Intergenerational trauma describes the psychological or emotional effects that can be experienced by people who live with trauma survivors. Coping and adaptation patterns developed in response to trauma can be passed from one generation to the next.

5. Historical trauma is a cumulative and psychological wounding over the lifespan and across generations emanating from massive group trauma. A subjugating, dominant population inflicts collective traumas. Examples of historical trauma include genocide, colonialism (for example, residential schools), slavery, and war. Intergenerational trauma is an aspect of historical trauma.

How many have you experienced __/5?

Transfer your comments onto your personal summary page.

With the state of the world today in 2022, and what we know about trauma, I believe the fallout will be catastrophic.

> *"Trauma comes back as a reaction, not a memory."*
> —Bessel Van Der Kolk

Lets look at how your brain reacts when it is traumatized:

Your brain on trauma: Untrusting; pessimistic; self-sabotaging; distracted; unmotivated; self-critical; judgmental of yourself and others and emotionally cut off.

Transfer your comments onto your personal summary page.

Trauma affects people, physically, emotionally, and spiritually. If you were very young when you sustained trauma, it would have altered your brain activity, as already discussed. You may remember traumatic things that have happened to you, and you might not. Trauma may have occurred as a young child and you were told not to tell anyone your "secret," meaning traumatic events may be disguised, however still caused brain alterations/damage.

When I sustained trauma at a young age, or as an adult, I didn't *physiologically feel* my brain change. I imagine if you could measure the effects of trauma in the brain, like a math equation, it would be seen as concrete but the treatment may be identified as urgent.

> *Addiction is not your fault,
> but healing is your responsibility."*

Unfortunately, measuring and treating trauma is complex. Personally, I don't know anyone that made addiction a choice. Think about it; when children talk about what they want to be when they grow up, I'm sure no one says, "I want to be a drug addict or I want to be an alcoholic," nor do they ask for traumatic things to happen to them.

> *"Cannabis isn't a gateway drug.*
>
> *Alcohol isn't a gateway drug.*
>
> *Nicotine isn't a gateway drug.*
>
> *Caffeine isn't a gateway drug.*
>
> *Trauma is the gateway.*
>
> *Childhood abuse is the gateway.*
>
> *Molestation is the gateway.*
>
> *Neglect is the gateway.*
>
> *Drug abuse, violent behavior, hyper sexuality, and self-harm are often symptoms (not the cause) of much bigger issues. And it almost always stems from a childhood filled with trauma, absent parents, and an abusive family.*
>
> *But most people are too busy laughing at the homeless and drug addicts to realize your own children could be in their shoes in 15 years.*
>
> *Communicate. Empathize. Rehabilitate."*
>
> —Russell Brand

My belief is that the gateway to addiction is trauma, and that's why addiction has been medically mistreated.

> *"Drugs have been around for a long time, so why are the "problems" getting worse? Could it be that drugs are not the problem, but instead a symptom of the problem(s)? Poverty, mental illness, lack of opportunity, disconnection from society, education, and poor laws. People need not be so naïve as to think this is just a drug problem; it is much bigger than that."*

In the next exercise, it may be difficult to recall every time you have been traumatized, so I encourage you to make your support person aware of what you are doing please.

In order to recall every time you have been traumatized, it will be easier to break down the events by grouping your memories on an age-range timeline starting with the present and going backward in your lifetime. Or, you can group your lifespan into groups such as childhood, pre-teen, teenage, 20s, 30s, 40s, etc. I also advise you to leave space to fill in more memories that may come back to your mind once you start to remember the traumatic events that you have endured.

Now, every traumatic event that you just listed needs its own heading and space below it to expand on.

I will list a few common traumatic events and create a template for you to enter your answers.

9. Abuse

Example event: Abuse

Your age(s) at the time of the abuse:

_____
_____
_____
_____
_____

Who was involved?

_____
_____
_____
_____

Where did it happen?

_____
_____
_____
_____

For how long did it happen?

_____
_____
_____
_____

How did the abuse stop?

_____
_____
_____
_____

Did you require medical treatment (physical and or mental) either during or after the event?

_____
_____
_____
_____
_____

If you received medical treatment for your injuries, do you have permanent physiological or psychological issues now?

_____
_____
_____
_____
_____

If you received mental health treatment how long were you treated for?

_____
_____
_____
_____
_____

Do you have the option of getting more treatment in the future?   Y/N

Were you able to tell someone, and if so, whom, or were you rescued?

_____
_____
_____
_____

Were criminal charged filed?   Y/N

Do you have contact with your abuser anymore? If yes, why?

_____
_____
_____
_____

Did you tell anyone that you were being abused?   Y/N

Did you have to hide physical injuries from others?

_____
_____
_____
_____

Did you start to physically hurt yourself after you were abused? If yes, what did you do? (e.g. cutting)?

_____
_____
_____

Do you feel that you live in fear now, having sustained that abuse? How so?

_____

_____

_____

_____

Do you isolate yourself or stop going to places you used to enjoy since you were abused?   Y/N

Do you suffer from PTSD (Post Traumatic Stress Disorder)? What is your treatment to help you with that?

_____

_____

_____

_____

Have you ever joined a support group for victims of abuse?   Y/N

Have you called an anonymous help line?   Y/N

Has your personality changed since you were abused compared with before the abuse? How so?

_____

_____

_____

Do you feel that you deserved the abuse? If yes, why?

_____

_____

_____

_____

Do you feel that you caused the abuse to happen because of something you did or said?

_____

_____

_____

_____

Was the physical abuse meant to control or punish you? If so, explain:

_____

_____

_____

_____

Was the abuse viewed as a "normal" cultural practice? Explain.

_____
_____
_____
_____
_____

Have you ever witnessed anyone being physically abused? What stays in your mind the most?

_____
_____
_____
_____

How did that make you feel?

_____
_____
_____
_____

If someone physically abused you today, what would you do?

_____

_____

_____

_____

_____

_____

_____

_____

_____

Transfer your experience(s) of abuse you have sustained onto your personal summary page, but if you it's too emotionally difficult, simply state, "yes" indicating that abuse is/was an issue.

Please take a short break if/when you feel overwhelmed, and call your support person.

Just so you know, your trauma is still valid even if:

- you never told anyone
- you can't remember all of it
- it happened a long time ago
- people didn't believe you
- you are feeling better now

- you didn't realize it was traumatic until later on
- you know people who have been through worse
- your life wasn't threatened
- it didn't develop into PTSD

> *"Trauma is perhaps the most avoided, ignored, belittled, denied, misunderstood, and untreated cause of human suffering."*
> —Peter Levine

Drug addiction is only one side effect of trauma.

> *"Don't let the hard days win. You're gong to make it. It'll be hard but you're going to make it."*

Feeling supported and free of judgment helps healing to occur.

Let's talk about anxiety and depression:

Anxiety is a feeling that challenges your ability to cope. It is a manifestation of doubt. Anxiety stems from trauma and stress, causing anxiety to be a trigger to use. "20 percent of Americans with a mood or anxiety disorder also have a substance use disorder, and about 20 percent of those with substance use disorder have an anxiety or mood disorder" (Carmona, 2022).

Depression and substance abuse are considered a dual diagnosis, affecting 75 percent of people (Polaris Teen Center, 2018). Whether depression comes before substance abuse, is similar to the question whether the chicken came before the egg—it can go either way, so the point is that depression is very common, and it requires treatment.

10. Anxiety

Taking a look at anxiety, let's answer some questions:

Do you have anxiety?   Y/N

If you have anxiety, do you take anti-anxiety medication?

_____

_____

_____

How do you feel when you're anxious? (e.g., mentally and physically)

_____

_____

_____

Do you feel uncomfortable with pauses in communication?   Y/N

Does your anxiety stop you from talking to family or friends?   Y/N

Does anxiety cause you to lose/miss time from your job?   Y/N

How many days per week would you say that you are anxious? _____

What are things that make you feel anxious?

_____

_____

_____

Do you wake up feeling anxious sometimes?   Y/N?

Please list everything you do to feel better when you are anxious.

_____

_____

_____

_____

When you are anxious have you ever called a help line?   Y/N

Has anxiety ever caused you to have to go to a hospital emergency room for treatment? When? How did that help you?

_____

_____

_____

_____

Whom do you call or want to see when you are anxious?

_____

_____

_____

_____

How does this person help you feel less anxious?

Do you feel an automatic response to want to use when you feel anxious?

Other comments about your anxiety.

Transfer your comments onto your personal summary page.

Ask yourself if you became anxious by recalling things that make you feel anxious. If it did, please know how important it was for you to do this. We have to "feel it" to heal it.

Take a break if you feel overwhelmed and consider calling your support person.

> *"You were not created to live feeling defeated, ashamed, depressed, guilty, or unworthy."*

11. Depression

Well done. Your answers are a vital piece of your recovery plan. Now that we've discussed anxiety, let's take a look at depression:

Are you depressed?   Y/N

What makes you feel depressed?

_____

_____

_____

_____

Do you take antidepressants?

_____

_____

_____

_____

How does depression affect your daily routine?

_____

_____

_____

_____

Does depression stop you from talking to or seeing family or friends?

Does depression cause you to lose time at work?

Does your personal hygiene get neglected when you are depressed?

Describe how you feel when you are depressed.

What are some things that make you feel depressed?

_____

_____

_____

_____

Do you feel depressed as soon as you wake up?   Y/N

List all of the things you do to feel better when you are depressed.

_____

_____

_____

_____

_____

_____

_____

When you are depressed, do you ever call a help line?   Y/N

Has depression ever caused you to go to a hospital emergency room for treatment? Were you admitted? Describe what you remember.

_____
_____
_____
_____

Who is the person that you call or want to see when you are depressed?

_____
_____
_____
_____

How does this person make you feel better?

_____
_____
_____
_____

Is it automatic to want to use when you are depressed?   Y/N

What is the first thing you reach for to make you feel better?

_____
_____
_____
_____

Is there anything else about your depression that you need to say/describe here?

_____
_____
_____
_____
_____
_____
_____
_____
_____

Transfer your comments onto your personal summary page.

I know that was a lot to unpack, so take a break, or reach out to your support person if you need to.

I dislike feeling like a victim of my own thoughts. It feels like a burden to have a busy mind and I feel like I'm "circling the drain!" When I am feeling anxious or depressed I ask myself whether the situation I'm upset about will matter in one week, one month, one year, or not at all. I try to put it into perspective because when I was in active addiction, every difficult situation felt extreme—needing more of me than I felt I could give. Categorizing difficult situations helps me to re-center myself and gives my mind the break it needs.

> *"When we are no longer able to change a situation, we are challenged to change ourselves."*
> —Viktor Frankl

12. General Questions

It's time for you to answer a variety of general questions below. This was designed to increase your awareness.

Are you ready? If you find your thoughts trying to sabotage your effort, take a short break and then continue. Be kind to yourself.

REMINDER: Being brutally honest will contribute to a stronger recovery.

In your own words...

What does illness mean to you?

___

___

___

___

List your illnesses or medical conditions.

___

___

___

___

___

___

___

Do you consider yourself healthy? Why or why not?

___

In your own words, what does it mean to be addicted to something?

___

What do you think you may be addicted to?

___

Is there alcohol and/or substance use in your family? If yes, name the relationship to you (e.g., mother, sister).

_____

_____

What age were you when you started using?

_____

_____

Did you use to numb your feelings? If yes, give an example of a situation when you felt it was necessary.

_____

_____

_____

_____

Did you use for fun?   Y/N

Do you have children? (If yes, names and ages)

_____

_____

_____

Did you use in front of your children or other family members?   Y/N

Did you use while at work?   Y/N.

Name 2 things you hate.

_____

_____

Why do you hate them?

_____

_____

_____

_____

What does it feel like to be supported by someone?

_____

_____

_____

_____

Do you feel supported?   Y/N

Who are the people that support you and how long have you known them?

How do they support you?

___

What is Love?

___

Do you love anyone?   Y/N?

Whom do you love?

___

Why do you love them?

_____
_____
_____
_____
_____
_____
_____

Whether or not you are currently in a relationship, name 5 things or qualities that your person must have for you to be happy and content/satisfied in a relationship.

1. _____
_____

2. _____
_____

3. _____
_____

4. _____

5. _____

What 5 positive qualities do you bring to a relationship?

1. _____

2. _____

3. _____

4. _____

5. _____

What is your source of income (employment, social assistance)?

_____

What are your finances like? Do you have any extra money at the end of the month?

___

What do you spend too much money on that requires cutting back?

___

Did you use alone or with others?

Have you ever tried to stop using before? If yes, when was that?

What is your longest period of remission?

Do you have a place to live?   Y/N

Is it safe there? If not, list your other options.

Are you fairly comfortable meeting new people, or is it a struggle?

___

Do you look forward to having time alone, or does that make you lonely?

___

What are some things you do when you're alone?

___

What kind of things do you like to do with others?

Do you have social anxiety? If yes, do you know why?

What motivates you?

What do you have control of?

What are your hobbies?

_____
_____
_____
_____
_____
_____
_____

Do you collect anything (e.g., memorabilia, coins)?

_____
_____
_____
_____
_____
_____
_____

Would you consider yourself sentimental? If yes, what about?

Do you enjoy listening to music?   Y/N

If yes, what kind or what genre(s)? (e.g., rock; rap; country).

Do you play an instrument or enjoy singing?

What are a few of your most admired songs?

48. Do you like to write or journal? If yes, how often?

_____

_____

_____

_____

_____

Do you enjoy drawing pictures, or coloring, sculpting with clay, painting? Please describe.

_____

_____

_____

_____

_____

Do you like to dance?   Y/N

If yes, how often do you dance per month (at home or out)?

_____

_____

_____

Do you exercise?   Y/N

If yes, describe your workout routine:

_____

_____

_____

_____

_____

_____

_____

Is it important to you to exercise to reach your best health?   Y/N

What other things do you do to keep healthy?

_____

_____

_____

_____

_____

_____

_____

Do you feel healthy right now?   Y/N

How many nutritious meals do you eat per day?

_____
_____
_____
_____

Do you know how to cook yourself a healthy meal?   Y/N

What are some examples of what you enjoy cooking?

_____
_____
_____
_____
_____
_____
_____
_____
_____

What season do you enjoy the most? (winter, spring, summer, or fall).

_____
_____

During this season, what do you enjoy doing?

_____
_____
_____
_____
_____
_____
_____

Do you star gaze or moon gaze? Do you follow astrology?   Y/N

Do you wish upon stars in the night sky?   Y/N

If you could be anything in the world, what would you be?

_____
_____
_____
_____

If you could have 3 wishes, what would you wish for?

1. _____

_____

2. _____

_____

3. _____

_____

Do you have any secrets? If you do, what are they?

_____

_____

_____

_____

Have you told anyone your secrets? If you have, whom have you confided in?

_____

_____

_____

_____

Do you have a favorite joke? What is it?

_____
_____
_____
_____
_____
_____
_____

Do you laugh out loud or do you chuckle quietly inside?

_____
_____
_____
_____

Do you like to go for walks outside?   Y/N

If yes, name 2 things that you look forward to seeing when you are out for a walk.

1. _____

_____

2. _____

_____

Do you enjoy nature? If you do, what specifically do you like?

_____

_____

_____

_____

_____

_____

Do you like animals?   Y/N

If yes, what is your favorite animal? Why?

_____

_____

_____

Do you have a pet? If yes, what?

_____

_____

_____

How long have you had your pet(s)?

What are the names of your pets?

What TV show(s) do you like?

What kind/genre of movies do you like to watch (e.g., action, drama, rom-com)?

Do you enjoy watching new movies or would you rather watch a movie that you have seen a lot and have even memorized some of it?

_____

_____

Are you competitive? If so, in what?

_____

_____

_____

Do you like yourself? Why or why not?

_____

_____

_____

How do you define right and wrong?

_____

_____

_____

_____

From these 81 questions, transfer your comments onto your personal summary page. Let's look in depth at the things that make you want to use.

"Addiction is an invisible attachment."

Attachment creates fear that gets in your way. Some examples are "what if I lose" or "what if I'm rejected," over and over. I recall an excellent YouTube podcast message about drinking: "I've never had only one of anything that made me feel good!" That is 100 percent true for me. Euphoria is addictive; we give great value to what we're addicted to. I idolized mine. How do you change that?

13. The Stages of Change

In 1986, Prochaska and DiClementi developed "The Stages of Change" to explain how and why people change:

1. Pre-contemplation: (no intention of changing behavior).

2. Contemplation/Preparation/A Thought: STOP!! DANGER!! (An individual will banter the idea of drinking back and forth until they succumb to drinking). This deadly thought accelerates into obsession (believing a lie) and couples with compulsion, in order to get your drink.

3. Ingestion: First Drink (the body is activated, and then craving begins). The body recognizes this and immediately has an abnormal reaction.

4. Craving: (happens only after the first drink).

5. Binge; Spree; Daily: Relapse (fall back into old pattern's of behaviors).

6. Shame; Remorse; Guilt.

7. A Firm Resolution to stop…repeats.

Don't forget — obsession overpowers any thought! Willpower alone doesn't work—not even *your* willpower!

The cravings, the compulsions, the need for more and more in pursuit of a high that offers less and less will not benefit you in any way. Being in active addiction feels like an insatiable thirst. Addiction is insidious. It's a bullet; fast or slow, it will *kill you!*

I used to find it exhausting to fight myself.

"Stop the tug of war—drop the rope!"

Can you recall when did your downward spiral begin? What was happening?

14. Powerlessness and Unmanageability

Have drugs or alcohol ever placed your life, or others' lives,' in danger? How?

How have you lost respect and/or reputation due to your usage?

What is it about your behavior that others object to most?

What will it cost you if you don't stop using?

List examples of what you have done in the past to fix, control, or change your using.

_____

_____

_____

_____

_____

_____

_____

Transfer your comments onto your personal summary page.

I've heard that you can't get fit by going to the gym only to watch other people work out! Same with addiction; *you* have to do the work!

According to the National Institute on Drug Abuse, recovery is 85 percent behavior change and 15 percent abstinence (Drugs, Brains & Behavior, 2020). When I initially read those statistics, I was surprised; I comprehend much more now and agree with that.

15. Ambivalence

Important information in *Drugs, Brains and Behavior: The Science of Addiction* reiterates how any change in behavior requires reinforcement and support due to the complexity of unlearning and then relearning. A barrier to this is feeling stuck, or ambivalent. Wikipedia (2020) defines ambivalence as "a state of having simultaneous conflicting reactions, beliefs, or feelings towards some object." Ambivalence kills.

"What you are not changing, you are choosing."

Recall a time when you felt ambivalent:

_____

_____

_____

_____

Did this negatively impact you? How?

_____

_____

_____

_____

Transfer your comments onto your personal summary page.

> *"Non-addict thinking:*
>
> *I burned my hand when I touched the hot stove, so I won't do that again.*
>
> *The addict tries the other hand."*

As with the stove example, why are we not convinced that using won't hurt us again? I don't get it. Similarly, why do we still think, in the back of our minds, that we can use again, even after being sober for a day, a week, a month, a year, or like me, 10 years? I still had unresolved trauma, poor coping skills, depression, anxiety, and denial, despite my clean time, because I didn't reach out for help.

As I reflect on that, I feel that ambivalence may have had something to do with my decision to not seek help. Part of me knew I had an addiction, but the other half was questioning it. The addicted side would remind me how great I would feel when I used and then craving would begin. As I have said, using begins with a thought.

Ask yourself if you are feeling ambivalent about having to work to do this work? Is there a tiny part of you that just isn't ready to put 100 percent effort into your recovery? It's vital to find out exactly what it is that holds you back, or relapse may well be in your future. Do you really want to take that chance.

> *"Don't let who you were talk you*
> *out of who you are becoming."*

What it is that stops you from being fully invested in your recovery?

_____

_____

_____

_____

_____

_____

_____

Transfer your comment onto your personal summary page.

You need to identify high-risk behaviors that can increase your chances of relapsing, like being around your environmental triggers. Consider this: if given the chance, would you get into the ring with a heavyweight champion?

No? Then why are you putting on the boxing gloves? Furthermore, why are you even at the gym?

16. Dangerous Thought Pathway

The first step toward relapse is a THOUGHT. The pathway is as follows:

1. Thought
2. Obsession
3. Use
4. Craving
5. Binge
6. Shame & Guilt
7. Resolution

Thought is a force that generates a physical feeling. I recall what I learned in rehab how "an obsession overrides any thought, so I choose to live in the problem or live in the solution." That's laid out in nice simple terms, but difficult to do. I had always thought that the first step to relapse was taking the first drink so this taught me to react much before that!

Working through your issues is a vital part of your recovery because your issues or stressors are what give you the THOUGHT to use. This is why you are strongly encouraged to work through every issue that haunts you, in depth.

During this process, the chant "let it hurt, let it bleed, let it heal, let it go," addresses the specific issue and work through it. This was another very effective tool I learned in rehab that helped me work through my issues when I didn't know how. I'm sure it's easy to identify your obvious issues: it's the sneaky ones that we forgot about that come back to bite you in the butt. This is where working with a professional helps you remember in a safe environment.

This is the reason I'm having you transfer your issues onto your personal summary page, so that it will help you identify what *you* need to work through.

17. Triggers

This brings us to triggers. I like to think of triggers as a big "Do Not Enter" sign! Triggers may be issues, people, places, or things that cause you stress, and make you want to use. You are the gatekeeper over what you allow to come in through your eyes and your ears, so be cautious.

Remember that people don't trigger you. They trigger your trigger. You are not your trigger. You are moved by your triggered reaction or activated response. Your trigger indicates what you need to heal.

List your triggers:

_____

_____

_____

_____

_____

_____

_____

_____

_____

"*The forest was shrinking, but the trees kept voting for the axe, for the axe was clever and convinced the trees that because his handle was made of wood, he was one of them.*"

—Turkish Proverb

18. Shame and Guilt

Awareness is the first step to change.
Barriers to change include negative feelings, such as shame and guilt, because they can keep you feeling stuck.

Dr. Kristalyn Salters-Pedneault and William Drake, (2021), describe shame and guilt as follows:

Shame — a feeling expressed by our thoughts, a feeling that you are bad, deserving of contempt, or are inadequate as a person. It is when you make a mistake that someone witnesses, causing you to feel humiliated or exposed. You feel powerless and this makes you feel weak instead of grounded. Shame is a feeling that replaces pride or self-esteem. I like to think of shame being the swamp of the soul! It's difficult to look someone in the eye when you feel ashamed.

Negative effects of shame result in having a decreased sense of self-esteem and a feeling of hopelessness. Shame may promote unethical behavior. I felt a tremendous amount of shame, having an image to live up to, professionally, but that was my inflexible ego.

Guilt, on the other hand is a feeling of remorse or responsibility for something you did wrong. It is an uncomfortable feeling to relax or to break your own rules or values. It is related to an act of wrongdoing, sin, or injury that causes us to focus on the feelings of others. What can you do to this situation? So, without obligation, make a commitment, take the initiative to resolve problems, and make the best decisions that you can. While some believe that guilt is easier to handle than shame, it still requires thought and effort.

To make things even worse, we stigmatize ourselves; this is also known as intrinsic (internal) factors (Deci & Ryan, 2000). Discrimination creates a huge impact when we lose the will to fight and, sometimes, the will to live. We became dissatisfied, restless, and non-compliant. Well, I'm happy to tell you that you can change this. Self-hate must stop. Your behavior is a product of "cause and effect."

It is simply your reaction to a dysfunctional event, not you personally. Stop letting your negative experiences dictate how you respond to your life today.

Has social stigma decreased your level of motivation to get help? Refreshing your memory, the definition of motivation is "a state of inclination or enthusiasm to change, which may vary with circumstances or time" (Motivation, 2021).

Stigma undermines motivation, as it attacks one's character and social class (Camp, Finlay & Lyons, 2002).

Additionally, stigma is a social threat to personal well-being (Deci & Ryan, 2000).

A person's motivation to get clean requires nurturing and support, not coercion. Social slander creates a sense of powerlessness and threatens self-motivation (Nagle, 1998). The consequences of discrimination are repression and cruel, inhuman degradation. Stigma causes many people to relapse because this destroys our new sense of dignity.

When others decide who somebody is before they get to know them, they take away the opportunity for them to be anything else. This causes those with addiction to feel 100 percent defeated, so they give up.

> *""We don't believe that cancer
> is a disease; we know it is."*

In summary, shame is described as a negative emotion and thinking, that we personalize, e.g., "I am bad. I am not smart enough." It sets invisible limits on ourselves and reminds us of our humanity and imperfection.

On the other hand, remember that guilt is a behavior. "I did something bad."

Do you have feelings of shame? Where do these feelings come from?

_____
_____
_____
_____
_____
_____

How do feelings of shame affect your life today?

_____
_____
_____
_____
_____
_____
_____
_____
_____
_____

What are some examples of your sneaky, dishonest, or deceptive behavior?

___

What do you do when you get caught in lies?

___

Whom do I usually hurt when I lie?

___

How do you usually deal with uncomfortable feelings?

19. Regret

Do you have any regrets? If yes, what are they?

What are some positive things you can do to move past your regrets?

What is your plan to stay honest?

_____

_____

_____

_____

_____

Transfer your comments onto your personal summary page.

To recap:

Shame attacks yourself causing a sense of worthlessness, and feeling something is wrong with you.

Guilt is breaking your rules or operating outside your own value system.

When you feel embarrassed, you own your shame.

When you change guilt into empathy, it kills shame!

Our emotions distort our perception, and it is this distortion that causes problems.

Unfortunately, we can be our own worst enemies and greatest critics, complicating our lives tremendously.

> *"Guilt is like crying over spilled milk—pointless and unproductive. Channel your regrets into change."*

When we were born, our personalities or ego formed based on how we responded to different situations. From our responses of how our choices made us feel, we ingrained specific values on ourselves. Now I challenge you to examine your ego.

20. Inner Critic

Consider the following definitions that describe the seven inner critics we battle with (7 Inner Critics, 2019).

Which one(s) do you identify with, from the most to the least?

1. The Perfectionist—tries to get you to do everything perfectly and attacks you if your work or behavior isn't good enough.

2. The Inner Critic—tries to control impulsive behavior such as overeating, getting enraged, or using drugs. It shames you after you use. It makes you feel hopeless, ashamed, inadequate, and guilty. You are in a constant battle with an impulsive part of you.

3. The Taskmaster—tries to get you to work hard in order to be successful. It attempts to motivate you by telling you that you are lazy, stupid, or incompetent; a demanding supervisor, or someone constantly multitasking.

4. The Underminer—tries to undermine your self-confidence and self-esteem so you won't take risks that might end in failure. It tells you that you are worthless and inadequate and that you will never amount to anything. It may prevent you from getting too powerful. It feels like "the rug being pulled out from under you."

5. The Destroyer—attacks your fundamental self-worth. It's deeply shaming and tells you that you shouldn't exist. It wipes out your vitality, creativity, spontaneity, or desire.

6. The Guilt Tripper—attacks you for a speculation you took in the past that was harmful to someone, especially someone you care about. Make you feel guilty for repeated behavior that it considers unacceptable in an attempt to get you to stop.

7. The Molder—tries to get you to fit a certain societal mold or act in a certain way that is based on your family or cultural morals.

It attacks you when you don't fit into that mold and praises you when you do. (e.g., a prison guard).

It determines what you should do at every moment.

Discuss why/how you identify with them.

_____
_____
_____
_____
_____
_____
_____
_____
_____
_____

Transfer your comments onto your personal summary page.

Again, please take a short break if you need one. Completing this accurately is vital—so don't rush.

Awakening yourself to your personality is steps toward understanding why you do the things you do. Identifying things that you need to work on is taking a giant step in the right direction.

21. Psychology Tools/Unhelpful Thinking Styles

Next, please analyze your own personality traits and love styles:

"Are you an avoider? Do you usually just say, "I'm fine" to try to get over it quickly?

Example:

_____
_____
_____
_____
_____
_____
_____
_____

Coming from often affection-less homes that value independence and self-reliance, the avoider grows up learning to just take care of himself or herself. The catch? They restrict their feelings and needs so they can deal with the anxiety of having little to no comfort and nurturing from their parents.

Are you the pleaser or the peace-keeper? Do you have difficulty confronting or saying "no" sometimes, making you less than truthful?

Do you seek connection and avoid rejection by anticipating and meeting others' needs?

Example:

_____
_____
_____
_____
_____

Pleasers usually grow up in a home with an overly protective or angry, critical parent. Pleaser children do everything they can to "be good" and avoid troubling their reactive parent. These kids don't get comfort; rather, they spend their energy comforting or appeasing their troublesome parent. As adults, pleasers tend to continually monitor the moods of others around them to keep everyone happy. Eventually, they become resentful and break down or leave the relationship or group.

Are you a vacillator? (Going back and forth, feeling insecure, and having internal conflict with high stress in relationships).

Give an example of your vacillator behavior:

_____
_____
_____
_____

Growing up with an unpredictable parent, a vacillator's needs aren't top priority. Without consistent parental affection, they develop feelings of abandonment. By the time the parent feels like giving again, their child is tired of waiting and too angry to receive. As adults, vacillators are on a quest to find the consistent love they never received as children. They idealize new relationships, but then get tired of it once life and the relationship gets less perfect.

Are you a controller? If you are, you are also very detached from your emotions, except for anger or happiness. You don't like being out of your comfort zone, and you make sure that you are the one in charge. Embarrassment is never okay. People describe you as intimidating.

Give an example of yourself as a controller:

_____

_____

_____

_____

_____

_____

Controllers need control to keep vulnerable, negative feelings that they experienced in childhood from surfacing in their adult lives. Having control means having protection from the feelings of fear, humiliation, and helplessness.

Anger is the one emotion that is not vulnerable, so intimidation and anger are often used to keep control. Control may be highly rigid or more sporadic and unpredictable, but controllers rarely realize the real reason they need to be in charge " (Yerkovich & Yerkovich, 2021).

Are you a victim? If you are, you tend to be anxious and a bit dismissive. You are fearful of being victimized due to so many traumas.

Give an example of your own experience as a victim:

_____
_____
_____
_____
_____

Transfer your comments onto your personal summary page.

> *"What would life be if we had
> no courage to attempt anything?"*
> —Vincent Van Gogh

22. Inner Child

Robery Burney M.A., who wrote "Inner Child Healing – How To Begin" (2002), discusses why there are feelings of inadequacy present. Your experiences may be based on your childhood or brought on by dismissive coworkers or managers or cultural theories. If so, you need to sort out what is yours and what others have made you believe in order to benefit them.

In chaotic homes, compliant kids survive by trying to stay under the radar and be as invisible as possible. They hide, comfort, and learn to be completely absent to alleviate the pain from their violent parents. Some children create a world in their head where they can escape the pain of abuse. Victims have no sense of self-worth or personality and often become anxious, and depressed. They may replicate their childhood home environment by marrying a controller and use coping strategies to keep them going.

A wounded inner child will feel inferior to others at the risk of serious rebellious behavior that is sometimes overly dependent and uncontrollable. A wounded adolescent will feel better than, invulnerable, perfectionist, needless, want-less and controlling.

We need to rescue, nurture, love, and heal our inner child and/or adolescent because if we don't, that child or adolescent will be making our adult decisions! (e.g., not leaving an abusive partner because you have abandonment issues).

Describe how your inner child/adolescent has been wounded.

_____

_____

_____

_____

Transfer your comments onto your personal summary page.

We need to stop our inner child/adolescent from abusing us as adults. How do we manifest that into our adult thinking?

Unhelpful Thinking Styles:

The following is a list of Unhelpful Thinking Styles (Whalley, 2019):

1. All-or-nothing thinking—sometimes called "black and white thinking."

2. Mental filter—paying attention only to certain types of evidence. Noticing our failures, but not our successes.

3. Jumping to conclusions—there are two key types of jumping to conclusions:

    a. Mind reading—imagining we know what others are thinking

    b. Fortune telling—predicting the future

4. Emotional reasoning—assuming that because we feel a certain way, what we think must be true. (e.g., I feel embarrassed so I must be an idiot).

5. Labeling—assigning labels to ourselves or other people.

6. Over generalizing—seeing a pattern based upon a single event, or being overly broad in drawing conclusions.

7. Disqualifying the positive—discounting the good things that have happened or that you have done for some reason or other.

8. "Magnification, catastrophizing & minimizing"—blowing things out of proportion (catastrophizing), or inappropriately shrinking something to make it seem less important.

9. Should/Must—using critical words like "should," "must," or "ought," can make us feel guilty, or as I already failed. If we ap-

ply "should's", to other people, the result is often frustration.

10. Personalization "This is my fault"—blaming yourself or taking responsibility for something that wasn't completely your fault. Conversely, blaming other people for something that was your fault.

Were you able to identify with any of them?

Rank them below according to which one you identify with the most, being 1, to the least being 10. Give an example.

1. _____

2. _____

3. _____

4. _____

5. _____

6. _____

7. _____

8. _____
   _____

9. _____
   _____

10. _____
    _____

Transfer your comments onto your personal summary page.

How did that make you feel?

_____
_____
_____
_____
_____
_____

Interesting, to say the least. Reading that made me sit back and reflect.

Take a short break if you feel you need to.

Now what are the signs of healthy thinking styles and what does it look like to have a secure connection with others?

- I have a wide range of emotions and express them appropriately.
- It is easy for me to ask for help and receive from others when I have needs.

- I can say "no" to others even when I know it will upset them.

- I'm adventuresome and I know how to play and have fun.

- I know I'm not perfect, and I give my loved ones room to disagree.

- I am comfortable with myself and with others.

- I am able to handle conflict, negative emotions, and both giving and receiving.

Furthermore, secure connectors are comfortable with reciprocity and balanced giving and receiving in relationships.

They can describe strengths and weakness in themselves and others without idealizing or devaluing. Good at self – reflection, the secure connectors clearly and easily communicate their feelings and needs. Resolving conflict was modeled for them growing up, so they know they're not perfect and can apologize when they are wrong. Setting boundaries and saying "no" is also no problem for a secure connector. They are comfortable with new situations, can take risks, and delay gratification. When upset, secure connectors create healthy boundaries between themselves and others.

Think about one reason why you might get angry. One thing that really angers me is when someone does something that they said they would not do. How do we protect ourselves from others walking all over us? (e.g., saying to someone, "It's not ok for you to talk to me like that.") We need to create healthy boundaries between others and ourselves.

23. Boundaries

"The shortest route to better boundaries is to really like yourself; better yet, love yourself."

~Unknown

A boundary draws a circle around you with chalk and says, "Enough!" An important part of our recovery is staying calm, and one way to safeguard ourselves from getting upset is to set down healthy boundaries around people, places, and things that we know are unhealthy for us, and doing this will promote this new version of you!

Boundaries are necessary to uphold healthy relationships, but beware; there will be individuals who are upset when you create boundaries because they won't be able to manipulate you anymore. Some may meet this with resistance and even try to make it look as if you are being unreasonable. Remember, it's difficult to predict how someone is going to respond to your boundaries. Be aware that you may have to readjust your boundaries in some situations, but adjusting your boundaries is better then abandoning them altogether. Abandoning your boundaries may lead to unhealthy behaviors such as self-hate, apathy, isolation, victim-minded, and using. When you think of the behaviors above, think about how you react when someone "crosses the line" you created. Those few examples are absolutely detrimental to your health and may lead to death if you use your substance of choice.

Boundaries need to be:

1. Rigid—tight boundaries, shut myself off/detach

2. Clear—what I communicate

3. Diffuse—applicable to different parts of my life

Let's practice. Name one boundary that you need to create between you and a family member:

_____

_____

_____

_____

_____

Name one boundary that you need to create between you and a friend:

_____

_____

_____

_____

_____

Name one boundary that you need to create between you and a colleague:

_____

_____

_____

_____

_____

Before you set out to approach all the people whom you need to set boundaries with, have your support person at arm's length, because you are bound to meet with some opposition.

Name one boundary that you need to make for yourself:

_____
_____
_____
_____
_____
_____
_____

What boundaries do you need to put in place for your recovery? Example: "I will not respond if I feel uncomfortable." "I will say no when I feel I need to."

_____
_____
_____
_____
_____
_____

Transfer your comments onto your personal summary page.

24. Trust

In order to set healthy boundaries, you need to trust that your decision is what is best for you.

What does "trust" mean, in your own words?

_____
_____
_____
_____
_____
_____

Andrea Bonior, licensed clinical psychologist, professor, and author, encourages the following actions for building trust as noted on the website *Positive Psychology—build trust* (Craig, 2021).

Trust is described as:

1. Being true to your word and following through with your actions and not making promises you're unable to keep
2. Learning how to communicate effectively with others
3. Reminding yourself that it takes time to build and earn trust
4. Taking time to make decisions and think before acting too quickly
5. Valuing the relationships that you have and not taking them for granted

6. Developing your team skills and participating openly

7. Always being honest

8. Helping people whenever you can

9. Not hiding your feelings – emotional intelligence plays a role in building trust

10. Not always self-promoting

11. Always doing what you believe to be right

12. Admitting your mistakes

Do you trust anyone? Whom do you trust?

_____

_____

_____

_____

_____

Why do you trust them?

_____

_____

_____

_____

_____

What other things do you value and need from those you trust?

_____
_____
_____
_____
_____

Transfer your comments onto your personal summary page.

Trust is a perfect segue into how we feel about ourselves in relation to our ethics and values.

25. Personal Values

It's important to know how you feel about your own personal values. Keep in mind that others judge us through our words, deeds, and behavior, so the following is a list is not exhaustive:

Rate these: 1=very important; 2=important; 3= somewhat important; 4=not important; 5=definitely not important

Value Score (1, 2, 3, 4, or 5)

_____ Accountability	_____ Positivity
_____ Achievement	_____ Entrepreneurial nature
_____ Adaptability	_____ Environmental awareness
_____ Ambition	_____ Ethics
_____ Balance	_____ Excellence
_____ Being liked	_____ Fairness
_____ Being the best	_____ Family
_____ Caring	_____ Finances
_____ Caution	_____ Forgiveness
_____ Clarity	_____ Friendship
_____ Coaching	_____ Future generations
_____ Commitment	_____ Generosity
_____ Community life	_____ Health
_____ Compassion	_____ Humility
_____ Competence	_____ Humor
_____ Conflict management	_____ Independence
_____ Continuous learning	_____ Initiative
_____ Control	_____ Integrity
_____ Courage	_____ Independence
_____ Creativity	_____ Job security
_____ Dialogue	_____ Leadership
_____ Ease with uncertainty	_____ Listening skills
_____ Efficiency	_____ Openness

_____	Patience	_____	Power
_____	Perseverance	_____	Resilience
_____	Personal contentment	_____	Self-discipline
_____	Personal growth	_____	Trust
_____	Professional growth	_____	Wisdom

Transfer your list and comments onto your personal summary page.

> *"Courage is the ladder on which all other virtues mount."*
> —Clare Booth Luce

Values or guiding principles need to be acted on, not simply stated. It's not "integrity" that encompasses a principle, it's "always *doing* the right thing." Expressing our values as actions provides a clear message to others and ourselves.

"There are several reasons why it is helpful to be able to identify your values because it helps you to find yourpurpose, helps you guide your behavior, helps you make decisions, helps you choose a career, and will increase your confidence" (Chowdhury, 2020).

Select your top 5 personal values and list them below, and be prepared to answer the questions below:

1. _____

_____

2. _____

_____

3. _____

_____

4. _____

_____

5. _____

_____

What actions display your defined values?

_____

_____

_____

_____

_____

Which personal value are you most proud of? Why are you proud of this?

_____

_____

_____

_____

_____

Which 5 personal values need to be worked on the most?

1. _____

2. _____

3. _____

4. _____

5. _____

Transfer any other comments on personal values onto your personal summary page.

When a situation causes a conflict between two of your personal values (for example career and family) what could you do?

_____

_____

_____

_____

_____

_____

How do you respond when you discover that someone you are speaking to disrespects one of your personal values?

How can I shape my career goals around what I enjoy doing?

How can I correct my values to ensure I will reach my long-term goals?

___

Transfer your comments onto your personal summary page.

> *"Your beliefs become your thoughts,*
> *Your thoughts become your words,*
> *Your words become your actions,*
> *Your actions become your habits,*
> *Your habits become your values,*
> *Your values become your destiny."*
>
> —Mohandas K. Gandhi

Let's take a look at your relationships surrounding love, play, friendships, purpose, and spirituality.

26. Love/Relationships

If you are currently involved in a relationship with someone whom you love (either friend, family, or intimate partner), why do you think there is a loving connection between you?

_____
_____
_____
_____
_____
_____
_____

What do you love about this particular person? (e.g., qualities; actions)

_____
_____
_____
_____
_____
_____

What do you think your partner loves about you?

_____

_____

_____

_____

_____

_____

_____

Are you positively affecting each other's lives? How?

_____

_____

_____

_____

_____

_____

_____

_____

For intimate relationships:

Are you satisfied with the intimacy you share?   Y/N

Examples of intimate things are: Familiarity; closeness; understanding; confidence; caring; tenderness; affection; relationship; quietness; seclusion; sex.

Which of those examples do you share?

_____
_____
_____
_____
_____
_____
_____
_____
_____
_____
_____
_____

Do their values match/complement yours or contradict them? How?

Do you apologize to your partner when you have made a mistake?   Y/N

Do you forgive your partner's mistakes? Why or why not?

Do you look forward to a future with your partner? If yes, why?

Transfer comments onto your personal summary page.

27. Play

Name 5 things that you really like to do/that are fun/that make you feel happy.

1. _____

2. _____

3. _____

4. _____

5. _____

Which of those five things do you engage in on a regular basis/routine?

If you do not do anything right now, how can you plan to do one or two regularly/routinely?

_____
_____
_____
_____

If you could do whatever you wanted for one whole day, what would that be?

Who are the most playful people in your life today?

What is the most daring/risky thing you have ever done?

What is your favorite childhood memory?

Transfer comments onto your personal summary page.

28. Friendships

What qualities does a real friend have? Do you have any friends with these qualities?

_____
_____
_____
_____
_____
_____
_____

Who knows you the best?

_____
_____
_____
_____
_____
_____
_____

What is the funniest experience you have ever had with a friend?

___

Has a "friend" ever suggested that you drink or do drugs with them, even when they know you are in recovery? (It happened to me, so be careful—expect the unexpected!) What happened?

___

What do you need to work on to strengthen your friendships?

Transfer your comments onto your personal summary page.

Keep this in mind:

If your friendships were developed during a time when you were using or traumatized, they are referred to as _trauma bonds_. Your growth means those friends can't emotionally attach to your weakness anymore because you are changing. Those relationships will reflect your past, not your present. I believe keeping those doors open will hurt you emotionally.

Suggestion: Take time now to reflect on every one of your friendships.

Which friends do not complement your healthy decisions or direction?

_____

_____

_____

_____

_____

_____

_____

Take action.

You may want to confront those friends and tell them to stop messaging you or simply do not respond when they message you—after a while, they will figure out that you don't want to have a friendship with them anymore. If someone disrespects your boundary, notify your support person immediately because this causes stress and you may need support to work through your feelings. You may have to consider changing your phone number. Do what you need to do to deny them access to you, or accept the consequences.

29. Purpose and Spirituality

What is the reason you get up out of bed in the morning?

_____

_____

_____

_____

_____

_____

_____

What is your life's purpose?

_____

_____

_____

_____

_____

_____

_____

What activities or ceremonies do you engage in?

___

Whom do I admire for their strong sense of spirit?

___

Do you want to create a more spiritual connection in your life?   Y/N?

30. Gratitude

Make a list of what makes you feel grateful:

If you feel grateful to someone, can you tell him or her how he or she makes you feel? Give an example of when you were able to do this.

_____

_____

_____

_____

_____

_____

_____

Transfer your comments onto your personal summary page.

Take a short break if you need to.

> *"Evolve so hard that they
> have to get to know you again."*

We need to be mindful of factors that can/will deplete our energy. Recovery is a time to rebuild your soul. Our souls connect us like an invisible thread.

10 Spiritual Secrets You Will Learn Over Time (VaderPack, 2020):

1. The sunshine is medicine.
2. Karma is real.
3. Prana (breath) is the life force of energy.
4. The moon strengthens your psychic abilities.
5. Everything is connected in this Universe.

6. Manifestation and lucid-dreaming is real.
7. Energies are real. Your body can sense energies.
8. Food is medicine.
9. Happiness and self-love is medicine.
10. Healing is an everyday process.

Things like feeling grateful and making apologies seem to begin to repair your soul. Being respectful, showing empathy, encouraging and helping others, respecting nature and most of all, giving and receiving love helps you feel grateful. Ego overpowers your soul when you are busy bragging or proving yourself. You may not realize that when you allow your ego to fuel your emotions and actions, it is destructive to your core.

> *"I still remember the days I prayed for the things I have now."*

Our souls are tired. We need magic. We need adventure. We need freedom. We need truth. We don't need more sleep; we need to wake up and live!

> *"The size of your problems is nothing compared with your ability to solve them, so don't overestimate your problems, and underestimate yourself."*

As you are recovering you will begin to realize that you are not the same person you used to be. The things you used to tolerate are no longer tolerable. Where you have been silent, you now speak your truth and you realize some situations no longer deserve your time, and attention. Choosing *how* to respond to something or someone involves your deepest thoughts from the knowledge you already have from experience.

> *"Just because someone throws you the ball, doesn't mean you have to catch it."*

31. Anger

Let's talk about the anger response.

The goal in learning about your anger is to gain knowledge about it and to learn how to control it. First of all, anger is completely normal, it is how we choose to deal with it that makes it positive or negative. No one makes you angry – you decide to use anger as a response. Anger is used and expressed in many different ways. For example, anger is a sign that something is seriously wrong; anger is used as an attempt to gain power over others; anger can also be used a means of survival in some situations; and anger is also used to try to find a solution to a problem. Notably, anger does not always lead to aggression – that is response chosen by us.

Here's another exercise. Let's take a look at an anger meter and then discuss the implications: 0 = no anger, 1–2 = starting to become angry, 3–4 = you are really angry, 5–6 = the point of no return, 6–7 = outbursts, 8–9 = furious, 10 = rage!

Looking at this scale, at what level do you think that you better do something about your level of anger? The answer is 1–2. This is the only stage that you will be able to control and intervene with healthy, calming things, or simply, remove yourself from the situation. Sometimes just taking a break to revisit the issue when you are free from anger will provide the ability to be able to work it out calmly and constructively. Does that make sense?

Let's answer some questions about your anger.

What makes you feel angry?

I get angry when I'm unjustly accused, when I have to wait, when others are inconsiderate, and when I am lied to.

Anger feels like a rush of fierce energy inside my body with nowhere to go!

Describe how you feel physically when you are angry.

Describe all the ways you express your anger.

Knowing how unhealthy is to explode, or suppress your anger, how can you deflect or calm yourself once you get upset?

_____
_____
_____
_____
_____
_____
_____

When does your anger become a problem for you, and what consequences have you faced due to expressing your anger inappropriately?

_____
_____
_____
_____
_____
_____
_____

Whom else did your inappropriate anger affect?

_____

_____

_____

_____

_____

_____

_____

_____

_____

_____

_____

Have you ever been a victim of physical discipline by someone in your family?

Child: Y/N

Adolescent: Y/N

Adult: Y/N

Comments:

How was anger expressed in your immediate family while you were growing up?

Have you ever been threatened with violence that might have killed you? (No names, just describe what happened).

Have you ever seriously injured anyone?   Y/N

What happened?

How did that make you feel?

_____

_____

_____

_____

_____

Do you have a criminal record for violence?   Y/N

Have you ever been to jail?   Y/N

How long were you in jail?

_____

_____

_____

_____

_____

Transfer your comments on anger onto your personal summary page.

Ok, it's time for another break. Please call your support person if you've been triggered!

32. Anger Assignment

It's time to do another exercise. Try this exercise every day for one week. Rate your highest level of anger 0--10 every day and write it down:

_____ Monday

_____ Tuesday

_____ Wednesday

_____ Thursday

_____ Friday

_____ Saturday

_____ Sunday

How did you do? What strategies kept your anger from reaching 10/10?

_____
_____
_____
_____
_____
_____
_____
_____

That exercise should help you to see whether you have some adjustments to make. What went "wrong" to bring on the anger response? In order to work through your anger issue, you need to break it down into manageable steps. To help you with that, Nina Maria Chychula RN, PhD and Cecilia Sciamanna RN, MSN help you to analyze your responses by breaking it down like this:

1. Identify the problem
2. Identify the feelings
3. Identify the specific impact
4. Decide whether to resolve the conflict
5. Address and resolve the conflict

Let's do an example:

1. The problem: My boyfriend got really angry when I went out with my friends on a Saturday night.
2. Feelings: Jealousy, abandonment, disloyalty, mistrust.
3. Impact: Dissolve the relationship.
4. Resolve: Break-up

It's pretty clear how anger contributes to unhealthy thoughts. Potentially, the alternative is using, illness, and death.

Conflicting feelings arise based on our relationship with the person we are angry with.

Here are some examples of how rules and messages may cause you to become angry:

- You aren't good enough!
- Don't express your feelings!
- Don't cry!
- Don't ask questions!
- Don't betray the family!
- Keep the family secret(s)!

- Don't contradict me!
- Be seen and not heard!
- No back talk!
- You are stupid!
- I promise (but breaks the promise)

Ideas of what you can do when you need help with anger, or with anything else mentioned earlier. Feel free to add more to the list below:

1. Call your support person.
2. Call an emergency help line.
3. Go to a hospital emergency department.
4. Talk it out with the person(s) involved.
5. Take a time-out.
6. Count in your head until you calm down.
7. Go for a walk.
8. Exercise.
9. Shower/bathe.
10. Drink chamomile tea.
11. Keep a journal/anger log.

Consider using this list as a screen saver on your phone, or write this out on paper for your purse/wallet for easy access when you need this in a crisis. It's very difficult to think when you're already angry.

"If you are still breathing, you have a second chance."
—Oprah Winfrey

33. Resentment

Let's talk about resentment. What does it mean to resent someone? It is said to be closely related to hate or contempt that is a generated from reality or from a perception of being unfairly hurt. "Resentment is a complex, multilayered emotion that has been described as a mixture of disappointment, disgust, anger, and fear. Other psychologists consider it a mood or as a secondary emotion that can be elicited in the face of insult and/or injury," (Resentment, 2021).

Resentment is self-centered fear that adds to the hurt and pain of an insult or injury. It allows others to control you and can follow this sequence:

1. Resentment
2. Self-resentment
3. Self-pity
4. Self-hate
5. Use (addictive substance)

Common reasons for resentment include the following:
- Being in relationships with people who insist on being right all the time
- Being taken advantage of
- Feeling put down
- Having unrealistic expectations of others
- Not being heard
- Interacting with people who are always late

—(Signs of Resentment, 2020).

Sometimes feelings of resentment are legitimate, but more so, have originated in your mind.

Let's answer some questions about resentment:

Are you resentful right now?   Y/N

If yes, what is the cause of your resentment?

_____

_____

_____

_____

_____

_____

What/whom does this resentment affect?

_____

_____

_____

_____

_____

_____

What was your part in this resentment, if any?

What are some ways you can end this resentment?

Do you resent yourself for your use? If yes, please describe how and why.

_____
_____
_____
_____
_____
_____
_____

Transfer your comments onto your personal summary page.

I resented myself based on shame, guilt, and ego.

> *"Resentment blocks the sunlight of your spirit,*
> *and dims your beautiful light."*

On a positive note, resentment can be motivating to set down some healthy boundaries against the source of your resentment.

34. Fear

Another block can be fear.

Write down all of the things you are afraid of:

_____

_____

_____

_____

_____

_____

_____

Transfer your comments onto your personal summary page.

My fears range from internal feelings to external ones over which I have no control. Fear is another form of self-defense that protects you or keeps you in a closed mind. I encourage you to discuss your fears with your support person in addition to writing them down here. I found that a lot of my fears were gone once I got clean/sober because many of them were just paranoid feelings caused from the side effects of the drugs/alcohol.

> *"Death from addiction comes way before the grave…"*

I believe grief is hard to deal with because the amount of love and grief are usually equal. Usually, the more you loved someone, the harder you grieve. The reason you never completely heal is because love continues to live on in your heart. You also make a new association: that persons' name with the painful feeling of the loss. For myself, when -I think about my late mother, the intensity of the grief hasn't changed; the frequency has.

35. The 7 Stages of Grief

According to Pacheco, (2018); the 7 stages of grief are the following:

1. Shocks and Denial
Most people react to learning about a loss with numbed disbelief. You may deny the reality of the loss at some level to avoid pain. Shock provides emotional protection from being overwhelmed all at once. This may last for weeks.

2. Pains and Guilt
As shock wears off, it is replaced with the suffering of excruciating pain. Although it feels unbearable, it is important that you experience the pain fully and not hide it, avoid it, or escape from it with alcohol or drugs. You may have guilty feelings or remorse over things you did or didn't do with your loved one. Life feels chaotic and scary during this phase.

3. Anger and Bargaining
Frustration leads to anger. This is a time to release bottled-up emotion. You may lash out and lay unwarranted blame for your loss on someone else, trying to control extreme overreaction, and permanent damage to your relationship(s) may result.

4. Depressions, Reflection, and Loneliness
A long period of sadness may overtake you. You might realize the true magnitude of your loss as it sets in and saddens you. You may isolate on purpose, reflect on things you did with the one you lost, and focus on memories of the past. You may also sense feelings of emptiness or despair.

5. The Upward Turn
As you start to adjust to life with your loss, your life becomes a little calmer and more organized. Your physical symptoms lessen, and your "depression" begins to lift slightly.

6. Reconstruction and Working Through

You become more functional and your mind starts working again. You will find yourself seeking realistic solutions to problems posed.

7. Acceptances and Hope

In the last stage, you learn to accept and deal with the reality of your situation. Acceptance does not necessarily mean happiness. With the pain and turmoil you experienced, you can never return to the carefree, untroubled you that existed before the tragedy, but you will find a way forward. You may eventually start to look forward and plan for the future. You may be able to think about your lost loved one in sadness, but without excruciating pain. You may be able to anticipate some good times to come, and, yes, even find joy in the experience of living.

How do we move forward when we are grieving? I can attest to trying to drink away grief, but it didn't work, not even a little bit.

John Pollard developed the following 10 stages of Grieving and Recovery (Crenshaw, 1995):

1. Acknowledge the loss.
2. Express your emotions.
3. Take time and make space—be gentle with yourself.
4. Recognize unfinished business (anger maybe).
5. Resolve ambivalence—and conflicting emotions.
6. Say goodbye when it feels right.
7. Commemorate the loss—rituals and customs to honor your losses.
8. Get out and get support—reconnect.
9. Meditate and exercise.
10. Forgive and move on—let go of "what if's" and accept your humanness, you heal and move on to new dreams, new hopes, and new lives.

I found it interesting how grief may mask itself in the following emotions:

Denial	Reflection
Loss	Hurt
Sadness	Distrust
Anxiety	Fear
Depression	Anger
Dread	Jealousy
Vindictiveness	Envy
Abandonment	Bitterness
Woe	Betrayal
Disappointment	Helplessness
Emptiness	Pain
Despair	Rage
Inadequacy	Sorrow
Resentment	Apathy
Anguish	Dismay
Regret	Panic
Relief	Confusion
Guilt	Loneliness

Needless to say, this list was longer than I thought it would be. Do the concepts of grief make sense to you?

Grief is a threat to recovery. Dedicating yourself to your recovery is non-negotiable. It is a matter of life and death.

The danger of addiction is there is no guarantee you will make it out alive. Some people are not given the gift of recovery in time. Three of my friends weren't so lucky. Their deaths are nothing short of a tragedy, because they could have been prevented. So, fight for your life while you still have one!

Whom have you lost to addiction? Are you currently grieving them? How are you dealing with it?

_____
_____
_____
_____
_____
_____
_____
_____
_____
_____
_____
_____

Transfer your comments onto your personal summary page.

The deadliest THOUGHT that has claimed countless lives:
"I will use JUST ONE MORE TIME."

Now that you have gotten clean and sober, you may be surprised that you aren't feeling as good as you thought you would. It may feel like your brain is foggy or sluggish.

36. Post Acute Withdrawal

You haven't lost your mind; you have Post Acute Withdrawal Syndrome (PAWS)

When most people think about recovery, they assume that as soon as you stop the drugs, your behavior changes and you are good to go. However, something that makes sobriety difficult is PAWS. "PAWS occurs in 75–95 percent of recovering alcoholics/addicts; symptoms appear 7–14 days into abstinence, after stabilization from the acute withdrawal" (Gorski, 2012). Post-acute withdrawal is a bio-psychosocial syndrome. It is caused by the damage to the nervous system that results from alcohol or drugs and the psychosocial stress of coping with life without drugs or alcohol (Gorski, 2012). Recall the discussion about how the brain is affected by drugs—although it regenerates itself, PAWS describes the time frame between using and being clean. I have to say that after detoxing, I really thought that I had suffered serious, permanent brain damage.

Symptoms of PAWS are the following:

- Inability to think clearly
- Memory problems
- Emotional overreactions or numbness
- Coordination problems
- Sleep disturbances
- Stress sensitivity

Transfer your comments onto your personal summary page.

The mental readjustment does not occur rapidly. Recovery from nervous system damage is usually 6 to 24 months. I was relieved to learn that PAWS does not affect intelligence. Yet, one of the most common symptoms is the inability to concentrate. As I said before, recovery is not linear, making it extremely difficult to adjust and readjust.

Additionally, memory problems are quite common, as your memory may become cloudy or may disappear altogether for a while. You might also feel "over emotional" because your emotions stopped while you were using, so now they feel excessive and uncontrollable. Focusing the mind is also especially difficult. Furthermore, you are often unable to distinguish between low-stress situations and high-stress situations. You may not notice low levels of stress, and then react excessively when you realize you have stress.

Most people have sleep problems, usually involving having bad dreams, but they do become less frequent and less severe as the length of abstinence increases. You may also have trouble with your balance, making you clumsy, because your hand-eye coordination and reflexes are slow. This is called "dry drunk" because you stumble around as if you were intoxicated. Since you can't remove yourself from ALL stress, here are a few suggestions of how to manage symptoms of PAWS:

Stress intensifies symptoms of PAWS, therefore learning to manage stress can help to control it. You learn to identify sources of stress and improve your decision-making skills and problem-solving skills to become stabilized. It is important to talk to people who will not criticize or minimize what you are experiencing. It's important to describe your experience to confirm your new feelings to problem solve and set achievable goals. This will improve your confidence. It is enlightening to monitor your progress. Try to think of this time as a time when education and retraining occur. Learning about your addiction, your recovery, and post-acute withdrawal symptoms helps to relieve anxiety, guilt, and confusion that would otherwise magnify PAWS. You need to learn management skills so that you know what to do when these situations arise.

Regarding nutrition, most of us were malnourished during active addiction. I lived on next to nothing to eat, and this went on for a very long time. The diet for a recovering person needs to include three well-balanced meals daily, and no sugar or caffeine. Hunger creates stress. Try to plan your meals and prepare them in advance. Caffeine causes nervousness and restlessness that often interferes with your concentration and your ability to sleep or stay asleep. Exercise helps rebuild the body while reducing stress. Exercise produces chemicals in your brain that make you feel good. These chemicals help to relieve anxiety and depression. Exercise reduces the severity of PAWS symptoms (Gorski, 2012).

How do you relax? Some suggestions include laughing, playing, fantasizing, story telling, reading, listening to music, and massage (Reiki & meditation), to name a few. There are a variety of relaxation techniques that you can try.

> *"Sometimes you can find heaven*
> *only by backing away from hell."*

How does motivation influence your stabilization in recovery? Change depends on your understanding of how you feel about changing your behavior. Careful selection, strength, drive, determination, and commitment are the motivating factors for an effective recovery model (Deci & Ryan, 2000). Self-determination theory, determines that human have three basic needs: independence, competence, and relatedness (Deci & Ryan, 2000).

37. SMART Framework

The SMART Framework is a simple metaphor that gives us clear, focused, and realistic goal-setting strategies: (Boogaard, 2021).

1. Specific: Define a clear, specific goal.
2. Measurable: Make sure you can track progress.
3. Attainable: Create a goal that is realistic.
4. Relevant: Ensure your goal aligns with the organization
5. Time-bound: Assign a target date to keep accountable

Let's do an example together and then you can do one that is specific to you:

Ok, my goal is to find a job at the grocery store, stocking shelves, within the next month, so that I will make money to live on.

S—I said where I want to work; specifically what I would be doing; and why I need this job.

M—the time frame (within one month).

A—I feel qualified, eager, and I have the transportation figured out.

R—This job will give me enough money to live on.

T—My deadline is one month.

Now it's your turn:

S _____

_____

M _____

_____

A _____

_____

R _____

_____

T _____

_____

Transfer your SMART goal onto your personal summary page.

> *"There is nothing more powerful than deciding
> to change your mindset and determining that
> you no longer will just wish things were different,
> you decide to make things different."*

Let's do a check-in and take a look at how you are spending your time.

In hours, how much time do you spend on the following per day?

_____ Working

_____ Sleeping

_____ Eating

_____ Personal hygiene

_____ Phone calls

_____ Text messages

_____ Emails

_____ Social media: List all accounts below:

Gaming:

How do you feel about how and where you spend your time?

_____
_____
_____
_____
_____
_____
_____

What other things generally occupy your day?

_____
_____
_____
_____
_____
_____
_____

Do you have any plants that you enjoy nurturing?   Y/N

If you don't have any plants, would you consider buying one?   Y/N

(A plant enables you to give love to something other than a person or animal)

What do you need to add you this daily routine?

_____
_____
_____
_____
_____
_____
_____
_____
_____
_____
_____
_____

You have been working very hard at this and it will pay off. Keep going! Time for another exercise.

38. Goal-Setting Strategies

Tell yourself 10 reasons to stay clean/sober.

1. _____

2. _____

3. _____

4. _____

5. _____

6. _____

7. _____

_____

_____

8. _____

_____

_____

9. _____

_____

_____

10. _____

_____

_____

"You're going to make it.
It'll be hard but you're going to make it."

39. Maslow's Hierarchy of Needs

It's common to feel mentally tired answering these questions, so take another break if you need to.

Let's answer a few more questions as we go back and take a look at basic needs.

The need to provide therapy to children from trauma and abuse is not new and it can't be ignored anymore! Children must be taught how to critically think and initiate healthy coping mechanisms to grow into psychologically healthy adults.

There are 5 basic needs defined by Maslow's hierarchy of needs:

1. Physiological survival needs (food, drink, shelter, sleep, and oxygen).

2. Physical safety needs (to feel safe in the world from personal danger and threats. Being deprived here results in fear. When a person is fearful, all concentration goes to calming their fear with no thought for any other task. For a person to develop fully as a human being, there must be some freedom from fear of personal attack (particularly in one's own home).

3. Love and Belonging needs (The need, and the hunger to belong to a group, family, religion, town, or class". Acceptance and understanding, loving and affection -- we need both to get and give love. Emotional intimacy is the need to share inner thoughts with others in close caring ways.

4. Self-esteem needs.

5. Self-fulfillment (self-actualization).

In 1943, psychologist Abraham Maslow developed his theory of human motivation in 5 stages and what he believed to be necessary for human existence and satisfaction. The consequences of unmet needs may develop mental health issues from infancy to adulthood. One of the consequences is "Addictions and compulsions, among 52 other issues commonly treated in therapy" (https://good-therapy.org/Maslows-Hierarchy-of-Needs/Common-therapy-issues).

Essential human behavior includes enthusiasm or longing for discovery, intimacy, learning, and protection. These requirements are necessary for all people for healthy development, participation, motivation, and well-being.

When our needs are unmet, it opens us up to unhealthy coping and relapse. It is vital to recognize your own warning signs to avoid a downward spiral because there is a small window of opportunity to seek help before using. For me it was as quick as flipping a light switch on, and then the craving would start.

Transfer your comments onto your summary page.

I believe that all people need their escapes from stress—some people engage in social media, some people submerge into a hot bath, and some people use drugs/drink. It's no wonder we need daily intervention in order to maintain our sobriety. Think about this: if you only eat only once a week, how do you expect to feel well for the other six days? Continuous support and connection with like-minded people is healthy a step that feels like a safety net.

> *"Recovery is not a straight line,*
> *that's why we need human connection."*

From what you have learned about addiction this far, consider the following:

We spend a lot of time trying to figure things out with your brain instead of your heart. Brain function created ego defenses and fuels relapse. It is better to consider trusting your heart, your good spirit. Your heart creates the humility needed to recover.

Recovery takes a little bit of mental energy however the key is to do so and to stay spiritually strong and connected. I heard something like that in a 12-step meeting and it was profound. It made me rethink what I thought recovery would require of me.

How did that make you feel?

___

"With equanimity, you can deal with situations with calm and reason while keeping your inner happiness."
—The Dalai Lama

40. Alternative Therapies

Cognitive Behavioral Therapy (CBT)

Cognitive behavioral therapy (CBT) is a specific, goal-directed approach for people to learn how their thought process contributes to their emotions and behavior. CBT is combined with techniques to help a person develop new constructive behavior (American Psychological Association, 2017). How often do you think about what you are doing at the time you are doing it? For example, right now I'm sitting at my desk typing on my desktop and there are several things running through my mind; go eat something, put on a load of laundry, etc. It is hard to focus on only one task at a time.

Mindfulness

Mindfulness is learning to live in the moment, instead of the past or the future. Right now is all we have.

Self-care

When you shower, envision the water washing away your fear, resentment, anger, and anything else that is causing your balance to be off. Water cleanses us inside and out. Other spiritual practices to restore your vibe include meditation (guided or silent), Reiki, crystal therapy, sound therapy, and music therapy. Having a routine of healthy activities to calm us makes it much easier when stress hits. Your body gets used to feeling this way, making it no longer automatic to upset our balance.

Reiki

Negative energy trapped inside your body is destructive and causes a sense of dis-ease, or disease! There are alternative ways that practitioners can balance the energy in your body. One way to release pent-up energy is through the healing art of Reiki. Reiki impacts us physically, emotionally, mentally and spiritually. [Reiki? 2016]

1. Physically, it releases tension and pain, assisting and increasing relaxation. Reiki benefits blood pressure, heart rate, anxiety, depression, grief, and anger, just to name a few.

2. Emotionally, Reiki clears heavy emotions to make room for more joy and pleasure.

3. Mentally it moves out negative thoughts that hold you back from being who you are.

4. Spiritually it connects you with your source of intuition and creativity.

This information was gathered from a 2016 article from the University of Minnesota's Baker Center for Spirituality and Healing called "What Does the Research Say about Reiki?" In this article, there are 44 references for practicing Reiki. It's not a new alternative therapy; it's just newer to the culture of Western medicine.

Meditation

Another relaxation method with positive affects is meditation. Meditation is the practice of quieting your mind, of turning off your logical brain. In our logical brain (left-side) we worry, we overthink, we stress, and we have using thoughts.

Meditation stimulates the right side where you think creatively, in an unscripted way. The practice of meditation takes you from the outside world into yourself. Take the time to get into a comfortable position (sitting or lying down), close your eyes, breathe deeply to relax, and listen. Some people may find it difficult to turn off their thoughts, or a song playing over and over in your mind, so there is another type of meditation that you can do. Instead, listen to a 30—60 minute narrated story, where you allow your mind go on a lovely journey. There are countless free meditations available on the Internet (YouTube). Meditation also provides benefits such as healing the brain by changing pathways. Meditation is an effective treatment for addiction, and is commonly done in rehab programs.

List the things you do to relax, with the exclusion of your addictive substance.

_____

_____

_____

_____

_____

_____

_____

_____

_____

Alternative therapy may help you heal your mind, body, and spirit. I recommend that you read about them, and see if anything appeals to you. Alternative therapies can help you to create balance in your life.

Balance

As I practice daily meditation and calming ceremonies, I feel balanced because I'm in a relaxed state. I'm more apt to "let things slide" and not engage in altercations. Consequently, I have learned how to balance my mind, and calmly get tasks completed, and not so much in a hurried state, rushing around. I'm able to listen to my body and my mind and take breaks when I need to, instead of pushing myself until I finish something completely. This is another reason why we are shown how to plan our day in intervals of time, to ensure that we are balancing our daily activities. I had to set an alarm every 90 minutes to remind me to change activities. Balancing my daily tasks is still not always easy, but I catch myself more often, and readjust.

Does this happen to you?

I'm going to use cigarettes as an example (nicotine drug).

Do you reach for a cigarette to "calm your nerves," when you get upset about something? I did. I was used to reacting instead of responding, and then tried to extinguish the stress with nicotine, a stimulant! When we feel uncomfortable, we attempt to change it immediately and this is a normal reaction, but we are not changing the stress in a healthy way, we are adding to it. I gave cigarettes all of my power. We are using a cigarette as a bandage; instead of confronting the cause, because our coping skills have been unhealthy. This is where you need to focus your attention.

Transfer your comments onto your personal summary page.

> *"Chin up, Beautiful. You're not struggling;*
> *you're in the midst of conquering."*

41. Connectedness

I was able to get clean and sober by utilizing a variety of methods and programs. Some people might get sober after they receive a frightening diagnosis from their doctor and quit using immediately, and some don't—the list is endless. Through aftercare programs at rehabilitation facilities to countless 12-step meetings in church basements and online, there is a lot of support already in place. It's free and accessible. Think about this: Knowing that MILLIONS of people have gotten clean/sober by building a 12-step program into their recovery, why wouldn't you at least look into it? One would think so but it's not for everyone. Some people dislike the mention of "God" in this program. So, perhaps you might want to try to reframe the definition of "God" to the metaphor—"*Good orderly direction,*" instead of the religious definition of God? It has been my experience that when we close--off our minds, it's a red flag. Maybe you are afraid for some reason? Don't be afraid to go to a meeting—the doors are open with caring people there who will help you get started and have walked in your shoes. Don't be shy. I have the utmost respect for the 12-step program, because it is a vital part of my recovery.

> *"I was always the black sheep,*
> *but I found the rest of my herd!"*

It's clear that connectedness is an essential key to relapse prevention; humans aren't designed to live alone. I isolated myself far too long trying to do things my way and never reached out for help. Think about it; if getting sober involved only willpower, we'd all be sober, wouldn't we? My peers are vital to my recovery because I have access to support when I need it. It felt so good to finally connect with others that have had similar life experiences.

These people understood me on a level that no one ever had before. After speaking with other people in recovery, I felt a certain connection to them. I didn't feel ashamed when I was with them because I wasn't being judged. At times, I actually avoided the mirror because I was too ashamed to look myself in the eye.

42. Honesty

This brings us to the concept of honesty. Being honest keeps our conscience clear, whereas being dishonest causes us to feel mentally overwhelmed as we make excuses—for using. It's a big hurdle for many of us in recovery because, let's face it, we had to be dishonest most of the time in order to keep using. We lied to everyone who questioned our sobriety because stopping wasn't an option. Being dishonest became so ingrained that we began to believe our own lies because we thought they sounded better than the truth. Lying is a trauma response. We also didn't see ourselves in the same light that others could see us in. Let me tell you something; they knew. They all knew. And I knew too. I came to realize that my mind was overtaken as I repeatedly chased the high. I was so mean to myself. I knew that when I used, I had only a tiny window of comfort, but the drug convinced me it was worth it.

So, how does dishonesty to others and ourselves affect us? We stay in a make-believe bubble. It feels protective, so we like it. Defending our words and actions make us justify why using is ok; it is a defense mechanism. I often thought that if I didn't admit to what I was doing, then I wouldn't have to stop. I knew that taking drugs and drinking was not good for me, but I couldn't deal with my life's mounting problems. I had the constant stress of my loved ones calling me out, which made it even more frustrating. I was fighting against my very own morals and values.

How does lying make you feel?

_____

_____

_____

_____

_____

The act of speaking your truth, or using your breath, is empowering and healing. It's vital that you are truthful, because if there is no truth, there can be little benefit from treatment. Admitting you have a problem and seeking help is a giant step in the right direction. Honesty produces trust and comfort, so remember that dishonesty is a deal breaker when we're looking for a partner or a business opportunity, etc., because, honesty is an attractive characteristic. Nobody wants to associate with a liar.

43. Morals

Let's go back. What is a moral? Google dictionary defines a moral in the following ways:

1. A moral is concerned with the principles of right and wrong behavior.

2. Morals are concerned with or derived from the code of behavior that is considered right or acceptable in a particular society.

3. Morals examine the nature of ethics and the foundations of good and bad character and conduct.

4. A moral is a lesson that can be derived from a story or experience (Moral – Google Dictionary, 2021).

Describe a time when you were dishonest and what the consequences were.

_____
_____
_____
_____
_____
_____
_____
_____
_____

Transfer your comments onto your personal summary page.

I feel it is important to love yourself. Make changes according to your needs. Progress or regress.

> *"It's not who you are that holds you back;*
> *it's who you think you're not."*

Now let us consider social stigma. People with addictive behaviors often have to deal with being told that they bring their problems on themselves. Furthermore, they are blamed for not getting them under control. It is ridiculous.

Here is a scenario that might seem odd, but it's food for thought:

Heart attack:
There are many causes of a heart attack; some factors are heredity, diet, and stress. Unlike other diseases, with heart disease our eyes can't see the plaque forming and building in the blood vessels around our heart. Hereditary factors are not a choice, and neither is trauma. This disease is silent until it progresses to a dangerous point. If the person survives the heart attack, they are started on a range of healthy treatments, and are monitored by their cardiologist at regular intervals to watch for warning signs of another heart attack. There is no shame, guilt, or stigma when others find out that you have had a heart attack. It forces you to change your daily routine in order to survive. This makes sense. There is also a lot of literature available to educate yourself, including many healthy alternatives. Now imagine how healing would be delayed or prevented if shame, guilt, and stigma were associated with heart disease. The paradigm would shift in an unhealthy way, making recovery much more difficult, in addition to being the epitome of ignorance.

We can agree that the complexity of our issues need to not only be addressed, but also professionally managed, and counseled on do you begin to find that? What are the options?

> *"Ability is what you're capable of doing.*
> *Motivation determines what you do.*
> *Attitude determines how well you do it."*

44. Symptoms of Stress

Do you agree that stigma causes stress? The following is a partial list of the symptoms that stress may produce:

Thinking and memory problems
- Poor judgment
- Inability to concentrate
- Seeing only the negative/pessimistic
- Diarrhea, or constipation
- Weight problems
- Skin conditions, such as eczema
- Nausea
- Dizziness
- Headaches
- Tension
- Chest pain
- Rapid heart rate
- Anxiety and agitation
- Racing thoughts
- Aches and pains of unknown origin
- Inability to sleep at night or sleeping too much
- Frequently ill — colds/flu
- Loss of appetite or comfort eating
- Irritability or feeling upset
- Feelings of anxiety
- Constant worrying

- Lack of energy to do things
- Symptoms of depression or general unhappiness
- Withdrawing from others/isolation
- Loneliness
- Feeling overwhelmed
- Procrastinating or neglecting responsibilities
- Excessive thinking
- Loss of sex drive
- Reproductive issues
- Frustration
- Feeling restless much of the time

Transfer your comments onto your personal summary page.

When you are hit with stress, please remember not to be too hard on yourself:
- You can be strong and need a break.
- You can be independent and need help.
- You can be kind and have boundaries.
- Some people have it worse and your pain is valid.
- You can do your best and learn more.
- You can be sure and things change.
- You can practice self-care and not feel guilty.
- You can be brave and feel scared.

*"You don't drown by falling in the water;
you drown by staying there."*
—Edward L. Cole

45. Myths About Recovery

Myths about recovery learned from my peers:

1. Life's problems will vanish once I'm clean/sober.

2. Others should be really grateful for my recovery.

3. Recovery should be easier.

4. It should be faster.

5. There should be no "should's."

"Let go of the illusion that it could be any different."

46. Daily Inventory/Recovery Checklists

Recovery Checklist Exercise:
The need to safeguard yourself is vital to your recovery. You need to work on your recovery everyday. A tool I found to be very helpful in my recovery was to keep track of my new and old behaviors by making a daily inventory checklist. A checklist consists of actions and responses that you can record daily. The left side, make a list of positive things and on the right side indicate the opposite. Put a check mark beside the behavior or action you took that day and evaluate this at the end of the month. The result gives you a good indication what you may need to work on. I found this tool to be very beneficial when I was in treatment (e.g., honesty _____ dishonesty _____).

Another important tool is having your own personalized Recovery Checklist of your daily routine.

Create another checklist with columns. At the end of your day, ask yourself if you have done the following healthy things for yourself and your recovery:

6–8 hours of sleep	Journal
Breakfast	Exercise
Lunch	Leisure activity
Dinner	Personal hygiene
Snack	Something social
Recovery meeting	Relaxation
Talk with your sponsor	Family time
Assertive behavior	Healthy self-reward
Expressed feelings	House chores
Positive self-talk	Job
Meditation	

The thing that I most liked about doing this exercise was being able to focus on me! It made a positive difference in my energy and in my mood because every day, I made time to do things for my health, instead of doing nothing.

It's vital to be able to identify what relapse behaviors are so if you are experiencing any of them, you will reach out for help: Relapse Symptoms/Behaviors – Warning Signs (Relapse Symptoms & Behavior – Warning signs, 2000):

Preoccupation: thinking a lot about drinking/using
- Irritability
- Impatience/restlessness
- Defensiveness
- Loneliness/isolation/avoidance
- Self-pity
- Dishonesty
- Neglecting recovery activities
- Resentment
- Anxiety/obligation
- Grandiosity/intolerance
- Self-righteousness
- Criticizing others
- Boredom
- Depression
- Poor diet
- Poor sleep
- Compulsiveness (spending, gambling, working, shopping, etc.)

List your top three highly risky situations that you may face causing you to feel like using.

1. _____

_____

_____

2. _____

_____

_____

3. _____

_____

_____

Transfer your comments onto your personal summary page.

47. Relapse Behaviors & Treatment

Relapse Symptoms:
What to do when you identify relapse symptoms:

- Get to a meeting
- Reach out to a support person
- Focus on your issues
- Do recovery reading
- Ask for help!! Get a Counselor/Social worker
- Express your feelings
- Journal
- Meditate
- Balance & structure
- Find stress relief by introducing some appropriate humor in stressful situations
- Exercise
- Do healthy activities—Fun/Play
- Eat and sleep well
- Avoid questionable people, places, and things (situations)

Transfer your comments onto your personal summary page.

List actions that you can take and do not appear above which are specific to you.

_____

_____

_____

"When times get tough, lean in!"

48. Relapse Symptoms/Emergency Tool Kit

Another tool for you to develop is compiling information that you will need in an EMERGENCY (when you are triggered).

You will need to list the following:

1. Support numbers: Phone numbers of people to call for support. List more than one and also include a helpline.

2. Reasons to stay clean

3. Consequences of using: List the negative things that happen to you.

4. Delay craving or Distraction tactics: List things you can do to ride out a craving.

It is vital to have this information at your fingertips 24/7 because it is almost impossible to remember what you need to do during a craving. I suggest putting it in a place that you will always have access to, you can make a screen saver or you can write it out and carry it in your purse or wallet.

After reading about relapse, do you think you can get clean/sober and stay clean/sober without any help or direction? No? Good. Neither do I. Don't get me wrong, ambition and willpower are required to plan your recovery but will not sustain it alone.

Finally, have a thorough *personal* recovery plan! You are actually beginning to develop *your recovery plan* when you transfer your comments onto *your personal summary page!*

Answer the following questions:

Where do you live, and whom do you live with?

_____

_____

_____

_____

_____

Are there any triggers you have where you live? If so, how will you deal with them?

_____

_____

_____

_____

_____

_____

_____

_____

_____

Are there any triggers where you work? If so, how will you deal with them?

Will you commit to recovery therapy (e.g., 12-step programs, other recovery-type groups)?

What support do you have in place and what are their phone numbers? I suggest putting their number in your "favorites" file on your phone.

_____

_____

_____

_____

_____

_____

_____

Do you have any social triggers when you go out or when you are on social media? If so, what are they and how will you deal with them?

_____

_____

_____

_____

_____

_____

_____

What other obstacles challenge your sobriety?

_____

_____

_____

_____

_____

_____

_____

_____

_____

Transfer your comments onto your summary page.

*"Slow and steady is my favorite speed.
I care about where I'm going, not how fast."*

49. The Addiction Crisis and Government Responsibilities

Addiction affects every level of society—from professionals to the unemployed. It doesn't care what level of education or job you have, or don't have, for that matter. The disease of addiction numbs your soul. Don't believe me? Just look into the eyes of someone in active addiction; they are lifeless.

It might be hard to accept that addiction is a life-long disease, but it is. Occasionally, the notion that you have "cured" yourself, may come to mind randomly, so you need to learn what to do when this happens. Immediately stop that thought, or you risk relapse.

The healing process is ugly. It's not all bubble baths and aromatherapy; it's accountability; it's getting to the root of your issues, which is triggering and intense. Processing trauma often means that you have to relive it. That isn't easy, but it's necessary. In a nutshell, you either want it or you don't. There is no in-between. If you want sobriety, you'll fight for it. If you want it, you'll find a way. If you don't, you will find an excuse.

Recovery is not based solely on abstinence from substances, but involves improving your quality of life in all aspects of your biological, psychological, social, and spiritual life. For the first time in my life, I put myself first, and refuse to be the people pleaser I once was. Now that I honor myself (and my recovery), I walk away from drama and negativity. You don't have to go to every disagreement you are invited to— so pick and choose your battles because you put yourself at risk when you rise to the occasion.

"Wear your tragedies as armor, not shackles."

What responsibilities does the Government have to combat the global addiction epidemic and prevent addiction in future generations? By providing comprehensive treatment— that's a starting point! Do you have an inpatient rehabilitation program accessible to you where you live? How much does it cost? Is there a waiting list? Can you wait? My friends died waiting.

I don't understand how treating the addiction crisis from the wrong end is helping at all. Clearly, safe injection sites, and the administration of the medication Naloxone (Narcan) to someone overdosing is not where to begin fighting the battle of addiction.

Don't misunderstand me, Naloxone is valuable; however, comprehensive treatment may decrease the number of times Naloxone is needed. I believe the government provides things like safe injection sites, etc., to make the public think that they are doing something constructive, when clearly it's not. It attempts to quiet the public, because it's cheaper than building enough accessible rehabilitation/trauma centers and programs.

I hate to break it to you, but the government is not only the gate, it is also the gate-keeper! They decide who gets treatment and who doesn't. That puts a price tag on rehab programs that most people cannot afford, nor can they afford to wait months and months to be admitted! There are many flaws in our medical system, but it can be corrected if there is desire or public alarm.

Our political representatives need a wake-up call, and we need to demand health care that serves everyone. To provide effective treatment, we must treat addiction from the beginning, not the end!

There are countless sources of statistics throughout the Internet reporting astounding numbers of people that suffer from addiction, from as early as 12 years of age, to the elderly. I'm unable to quote exact statistics, however, millions and millions of people suffer from this disease globally; and it is predicted that these numbers will increase dramatically due to the trauma of the global pandemic.

Residential Treatment Centers are available but only if you can afford to pay thousands of dollars to get in. Furthermore, detoxification costs are also thousands of dollars, so even if you can't afford rehab, you probably still can't afford safe medical detoxification. It's a catch 22. Granted, some insurance companies may fund part of the cost, but you will be put on a waiting list.

Luckily, there are a few non-profit organizations that provide free rehab for people in need, in addition to extremely limited free government rehabs in the USA and Canada, but that's better than nothing I guess. All I know is that society can do a lot better than this!

> *"Maybe if Greta Thunberg were an addict, governments around the world would initiate a comprehensive approach to treat the addiction crisis."*

We need programs that treat people of all ages for the traumatic events they have endured. Unfortunately, programs are not fully funded when there is no perceived economic profit. I challenge that by projecting the cost savings of treating trauma and addiction far out-weigh the cost of development. Astounding statistics indicate billions (almost one trillion) dollars annually is spent on related costs of addiction. It's only ethical to treat all of the people who suffer from addiction, not a select few.

When you are treated for addiction, you are also being treated for trauma, anxiety, depression, Post Traumatic Stress Disorder, rage, despair, and the list goes on. That's a tall order for 30-day rehab programs, isn't it?

Using a substance is often someone's best attempt to cope when they don't see other options with trauma-related stress. Children and youth develop unhealthy coping mechanisms from trauma, despite their best efforts. They are just not equipped. The problem with that is it becomes a pattern for the child, but now as adults, guess what? They haven't healed from their past trauma, and don't know how to cope with dilemma in a healthy way. It's not surprising to learn that in 2014, "90 percent of women in treatment for alcohol problems at 5 Canadian Residential Treatment Centers indicated abuse-related trauma as a child or adult; 60 percent indicated other forms of trauma. Furthermore, 90 percent of females and 62 percent of male youths in co-occurring disorders treatment at CAMH (Center for Addictions and Mental Health) endorsed concerns with traumatic distress" (Understanding Trauma, 2014). Government officials must do more to provide the means necessary to address mental health and addiction services for more than 30 days. Compassionate and comprehensive treatment for all ages is crucial.

But how does an individual, who just got sober, deal with future hardship without a safety net? People need to maintain connections and regular lifelong coaching.

To recap, there are countless research studies that indicate a correlation between substance abuse/use and trauma. Even with decades of indisputable data, yet, here we are.

There are not enough Residential Treatment Centers or professional outpatient programs available. That's nothing new. A delayed admission to treatment is the difference between life-and-death for many suffering from active addiction. Where is the public excitement? If something threatens the economy, it's immediately addressed. In other words, the driving motive is not human suffering, but profit and loss, which is the fundamental platform of our society.

50. Alcohol

This brings me to the matter of alcohol consumption.

The History of Alcohol

The history of drinking alcohol dates back 80 million years. Alcohol existed in early Egyptian civilization. Alcohol played a pivotal role in early Greek religious culture and was often used as an offering to the Gods (Villa, 2021). In the sixteenth century, alcohol was largely used for medicinal purposes, and by the eighteenth century, alcoholism became widespread. 1920 brought a push toward prohibition but it was cancelled.

I'm intrigued that the prohibition of alcohol was cancelled, as I ponder what documented factors and statistics led tothe call for prohibition. One big factor was domestic violence.

The Temperance Movement

"The Temperance Movement began in the early eighteen hundreds sought to reduce alcohol consumption due to the harmful effects of drinking to excess. By the eighteen twenties, members pushed for a total alcohol abstinence. People joining this movement became part of the *Cold Water Army.* The movement served both religious and social purposes, as some people strived to achieve societal and individual reform. In 1919, *The Volstead Act* specified that alcohol could only be produced or sold for medical or religious reasons, and it could only be consumed in one's home if bought legally. However, prohibition did not ban the actual consumption of alcohol. Many Americans purchased and drank it in speakeasies and with the help of organized crime. In the early 1930's, many believed that legalizing alcohol would help *boost the economy*, and the 21st Amendment ended Prohibition in 1933" (Villa, 2021).

It is my strong opinion that the selling of alcohol needs to be revisited. The time is now. Ask yourself: what exactly are the benefits of alcohol? The detriments are that brain activity is depressed and this leads to distorted decision-making, and impaired motor coordination. Statistics prove that millions of people suffer from alcoholism, and that fact is documented globally. Why then is it so accessible "e.g., sold in the grocery stores"? *It's revenue at the expense to your health.*

Effects of Alcohol on Society
Do the benefits of alcohol outweigh the risks?

"240 million people around the world use alcohol problematically" (Substance Use and Addiction, 2021). Alcohol needs to be prohibited again. It's a "no-brainer." The problem seems to be the sweet profit of millions of dollars that alcohol generates for government(s). Prohibiting alcohol would be quite a financial loss for businesses that rely on this revenue. Additionally, alcohol is threaded through the media, and it is socially acceptable. I recall when cigarettes were proven to cause cancer. The public concern/outcry was heard. The government banned smoking advertisements. It also published photos of blackened lungs and put warning labels on all of the cigarette packages. The same things that have been done against cigarettes can be done against alcohol.

> *"Let's start putting photos of people in active addiction on every bottle of alcohol."*

Advertising the glorification of drugs, alcohol, sex, food, gambling, etc., is the recipe for disaster in impressionable minds.

What are your thoughts on alcohol prohibition?

_____
_____
_____
_____
_____

51. Conclusion

I recall feeling very empowered after reading the following excerpt from Sharon Stone's acceptance speech after receiving the Woman of the Year award, 2019, as I could relate:

> *"Each and everyone of you will have a defining moment, a moment that changes your life. You might be aware of it when it's happening and you might not. But I'll tell you this: you're going to have one if you haven't had one already… and you're going to be held accountable for it, if you haven't already. And people are going to ask you a lot of questions, if they haven't already. So, the time to decide who you are is now! The time to decide what to do with the tender, important, beautiful, savage, passionate, most important parts of yourself is now! What are you going to do with it?"*

In summary, I'd like to leave you with this:

What I have lost in the last few years:

    I lost a partner, 2009

    I lost my dog, 2016

    I lost 2 friends, 2016

    I lost another 2 friends, 2017

    I lost a partner, 2017

    I lost my home, 2017

    I lost my mother, 2018

    I lost my relationship with my sister, 2018

    I got sober 6 months before my mother passed, thank God.

There is no way I could have cared for my mother and laid her to rest if I had been using.

So, I've told you what I lost. Now let's talk about what I gained:

> I gained knowledge of who I am, how I function, and why I'm here.
>
> I regained my ability to think critically.
>
> I gained respect for myself.
>
> I gained time.
>
> I regained the trust of my family.
>
> I gained strength.
>
> I gained the ability to form deep and lasting bonds with new friends.
>
> I gained the ability to love myself.
>
> I gained the ability to give and receive.
>
> I gained the ability to set healthy boundaries.
>
> I gained the ability to say no without the pressure to explain why.
>
> I gained clarification.
>
> I gained freedom.
>
> I gained the voice of spirit.

Yes, I still have tough times but I'm able to handle it, because I'm no longer alone.

> *"Be careful judging that drug addict so harshly...they may just recover and be the one to show someone you know a way out someday."*

I sincerely hope that this workbook has helped you.

If you think that you have a problem with substance dependency, please reach out and get help.

Let go of the illusion that your addiction is a mirage.

This isn't a disease that you can be passive about; it can kill you.

52. I Am Your Disease

You know who I am; you've called me your friend.
Wishes of misery and heartache I send.
I want only to see that you're brought to your knees.
I'm the devil inside of you; I am your disease.
I'll invade all your thoughts; I'll take hostage your soul.
I'll become your new master, in total control.
I'll maim your emotions; I'll run the whole game
Till your entire existence is crippled with shame.
When you call me I come, sometimes in disguise.
Quite often I'll take you by total surprise.
But take you I will, and just as you've feared.
I'll want only to hurt you, with no mercy spared.
If you have your own family, I'll see it's destroyed.
I'll steal every pleasure in life you've enjoyed.
I'll not only hurt you, I'll kill if I please.
I'm your worst nightmare; I am your disease.
I bring self-destruction, but still you can't tell.
I'll sweep you through heaven, then drop you in hell.
I'll chase you forever, wherever you go
And when I catch you, you won't even know.
I'll sometimes lie silent, just waiting to strike.
What's yours becomes mine, cuz I take what I like.
I'll take all you own and I won't care who sees.
I'm your constant companion; I am your disease.
If you have any honor, I'll strip it away.
You'll lose all your hope and forget how to pray.
I'll leave you in darkness, while blindly you stare.
I'll reduce you to nothing, and won't even care.
So, don't take for granted my powers sublime.
I'll bend and I'll break you, time after time.
I'll crumble your world with the greatest of ease.

I'm that madman inside you; I am your disease.
But today I'm real angry, you want to know why?
I let this treatment center full of addicts entirely slip by.
How did I lose you? Where did I go wrong?
One minute I had you, then, next, you were gone.
You just can't dismiss all the good times we've shared.
When you were alone, wasn't it I who appeared?
When you sold those possessions you knew you would need,
Wasn't I the first one who stepped in and agreed.
Now look at you bastards, you're all thinking clear.
You escaped with your lives when you found your way here.
Only fools think they're winners when admitting defeat.
It's what you must say when you're claiming that seat.
Go ahead and surrender, if that's what you choose.
But, I'm not giving up, cuz I can't stand to lose.
So stand in your groups and support hand in hand.
Better choices will save you, leaving me to be damned.
Well, be damned all you people seeking treatment each week.
Be damned inner strength, however unique.
Be damned all your sayings, be damned your clichés.
Be damned every addict, who back to me strays.
For I know it will happen, I've seen it before.
Those who love misery will crawl back for more.
So take comfort in knowing, I'm waiting right here.
But next time around, you'd just better beware.
You think that you're stronger or smarter this time.
There isn't a mountain or hill you can't climb.
Well if that's what you're thinkin', you ain't learned a thing.
I'll still knock you silly if you step back into my ring.
But you say you've surrendered, so what can I do?
It's so sad in a way; I had big plans for you.
Creating your nightmare for me was a dream.
I'm sure gonna miss you, we made quite a team.

So please don't forget me, I won't forget you.
I'll stand by your side watching all that you do.
I'm ready and waiting, so call if you please.
I won't let you forget me; I am your disease.

—The Haynes Clinic.com

53 Your Personal Summary Page(s)

1. DSM-IV Questionnaire score __/11

What came to your mind when you were reading these questions? How did it make you feel?

Comments:

2. **DAST-10 Questionnaire score __/10**

What came to your mind when you were reading these questions? How did it make you feel?

Comments:

3. Johns Hopkins Addiction Questionnaire score ___/20

What came to your mind when you were reading these questions? How did it make you feel?

Comments:

4. Alcohol Withdrawal Questionnaire score __/8

What came to your mind when you were reading these questions? How did it make you feel?

Comments:

5. Opiate Withdrawal Questionnaire score ___/10

What came to your mind when you were reading these questions? How did it make you feel?

Comments:

6. List the behaviors and personality characteristics you had when you were in active addiction:

Comments:

7. Trauma type:

What came to your mind, and how did it make you feel?

Comments:

8. Abuse:

What came to your mind, and how did it make you feel?

Comments:

_____

_____

_____

_____

_____

_____

_____

_____

_____

_____

_____

_____

_____

_____

_____

_____

_____

_____

9. Anxiety:

What came to your mind, and how did it make you feel?

Comments:

10. Depression:

What came to your mind, and how did it make you feel?

Comments:

11. Of the 81 questions', comment on those questions you had issues with.
What came to mind and how did it make you feel?

Comments:

12. Powerlessness and unmanageability: (your main reasons for using).

What came to your mind, and how did it make you feel?

Comments:

13. Ambivalence:

What came to your mind, and how did it make you feel?

Comments:

14. Triggers

What came to your mind, and how did it make you feel?

Comments:

15. Shame & Guilt:

What came to your mind, and how did it make you feel?

Comments:

16. Regret:

What came to your mind, and how did it make you feel?

Comments:

17. Inner Critic:

What came to your mind, and how did it make you feel?

Comments:

18. Personality Traits:

What came to your mind, and how did it make you feel?

Comments:

19. Inner Child:

What came to your mind, and how did it make you feel?

Comments:

20. Inner Child/Adolescent Issues:

What came to your mind, and how did it make you feel?

Comments:

21. Boundaries:

What boundaries must you set for your health and happiness?

Comments:

22. Trust:

What came to your mind, and how did it make you feel?

Comments:

23. Personal values:

What are your personal values?

Comments:

24. Personal goals:

What are your personal goals? It's important to list every goal you have, not just some (listing sets an intention).

Comments:

_____

_____

_____

_____

_____

_____

_____

_____

_____

_____

_____

_____

_____

_____

25. Love Relationships:

Who came to your mind? Why? How did it make you feel when you thought of that love relationship?

Comments:

26. Play:

What came to your mind, and how did it make you feel?

Comments:

27. Friendships:

What came to your mind, and how did it make you feel?

Comments:

28. Purposes and Spirituality:

What came to your mind, and how did it make you feel?

Comments:

29. Gratitude:

What came to your mind, and how did it make you feel?

Comments:

30. Anger:

What came to your mind, and how did it make you feel?

Comments:

31. Resentment:

What came to your mind, and how did it make you feel?

Comments:

32. Fear:

What came to your mind, and how did it make you feel?

Comments:

33. Grief:

What came to your mind, and how did it make you feel?

Comments:

34. Post Acute Withdrawal Syndrome -- PAWS:

What came to your mind, and how did it make you feel?

Comments:

35. SMART Goals:
Comments:

S _____

_____

M _____

_____

A _____

_____

R _____

_____

T _____

_____

36. Goal Setting Strategies

Comments:

37. Alternative Therapies:

Are there any alternative therapies you do now or would like to try?

Comments:

38. Connectedness:

Comments:

39. Honesty:
Comments:

40. Morals:

Comments:

41. Stigma/Stress
Comments:

42. Relapse Symptoms:

Comment on relapse symptoms you have experienced.

Comments:

54. Your Health & Personal Recovery Plan

How are you going to address each of your challenges to empower yourself?

Begin by prioritizing the challenges you need to work on right away.

This plan is tailored to suited *you*! (e.g., "Numbers 6, 8, 11 and 16 are my most challenging issues," and begin with those below). e.g., Depression:

> I'm going to talk to my support person – the person I trust, and open up to them; tell them why you feel depressed.
>
> I'm going to make an appointment with a doctor to discuss my depression, with my support person, and seek treatment because I know that I don't have to suffer in silence anymore.
>
> I'm willing to do talk therapy and try medication to treat depression – I will follow my doctor's treatment plan.
>
> I'm going to get outside for 15 minutes/day and breathe fresh air.
>
> I can go for a walk.
>
> I can do something that I enjoy doing e.g. gaming, reading, crafts, music etc. for 1 hour per day, to get out of your head.
>
> I can play with my pet…

_____

_____

_____

_____

_____

55. My Story

I was born in 1963. I have one older sister. My late mother was an RN and my father is a drafter. Growing up was fairly unremarkable when it came to alcohol or drug exposure. We lived in the northwest side of Toronto in a nice home. We were comfortable—not rich, not poor. I'm a third generation Canadian with Italian, Scottish, Welsh roots. I had no problem making friends and I was active in sports. Academically, I thrived in school. My parents emphasized how important education was and were very supportive of this.

The first traumatic event that I can recall was when I was about 7 years old and was playing near the road where we lived. A man stopped his car and attempted to abduct me by luring me closer to his car with a question. Thankfully my sister ran for my mother and the man sped away. I remember being told that the man could have taken me, hurt me, or worse, and I would never see my family again! That was traumatic!

Then when I was 10 years old, my parents rented a cottage along Lake Huron. One day we went to the beach—it was overcast, windy, and the water was a little rough. My father and I went out on the raft to have some fun in the waves. Long story short, I flipped off the raft and started to drown because I didn't know which way was up! Dad found me and saved me! When we were back on the beach, a few people gathered around us. The comments really scared me, hearing someone say my father saved my life! The shock was so powerful physically and emotionally, that I developed an immediate stuttering problem. Sadly, the stuttering didn't stop, so when I returned to school in September I required 1:1 speech therapy classes.

That year (Grade 5), I was teased and bullied by two boys, just to make things worse. They would pin me down on the playground and choke me! It was terrifying!! They chased me home every day. Thankfully, it stopped when I told my big sister and her friend. I reluctantly had to tell my mother, because I was petrified that the bullying would get worse. Anyway, my mother spoke to the principal, and the bullying completely stopped, thank God. Later, I found out that I was being bullied because one of the boys liked me. That was quite a mixed message of how a boy would treat you if he liked you!

One year later, my father was forced to leave my mother due to her mental illness. It was a shock to my sister and I because my parents never fought or argued in front of us.

Regardless of the reason, I felt scared and vulnerable without my father in the house. I was trying to process all of that in addition to my father's lady friend. Cat-calls about this lady were regular from my mother and her side of the family. In fact, that confused me because I liked her when I met her, but I wasn't supposed to. I blamed her for everything (that changed as I matured).

My father was, and still is, my mentor, my rock, and my greatest support.

It was customary to go to my grandparents' house on Christmas Eve. My parents' rarely drank, with the exception of Christmas Eve. I recall seeing my father have one drink with my grandfather and my uncles. Alcohol was viewed as a special occasion beverage for the adults. Period. My mother and aunts occasionally enjoyed a glass of wine. It was well known, in our family, that children didn't drink alcohol, or coffee for that matter. Those were the rules. Again, no one got drunk.

I was told that my great-grandfather was an alcoholic on my father's side. One of my great-uncles was an alcoholic, and a few of my cousins were alcoholic/addicts, and gamblers on my mother's side.

My first experience with strong pain medication was at age 16 when I had to have my wisdom teeth surgically removed. I was prescribed an opiate. This was my first drug-induced euphoric feeling! As I was nearing the end of the prescription I tried to get more, but was denied. That was my first drug seeking experience. Why did I crave these pills after one short week? Do you see where this is going?

Then, turning 19 years old was like getting the green light to drink because it was the legal age. I would occasionally have a few drinks or a toke at a party on weekends. Social binge drinking was normal and accepted among my group of friends. It seemed pretty tame.

In 1985 I started college to be an RN. In those days, nurses were told not to show their emotions to their patients because it was considered "unprofessional." Unfortunately this conditioning filtered into my personal life, leading to the habitual concealment of negative feelings.

I have been married twice.

One of my husbands was narcissistic and abusive, allegedly (according to what has been claimed).

I sustained injuries in a car accident and I required prescription medication to manage my pain. Unfortunately, I became addicted to the pills. The addiction created a dilemma because I had to return to work feeling less than 100 percent, or so I thought. The impact of that relationship, in addition to being medicated, clearly affected my decision making skills. I struggled with the physical requirements of my job, and eventually took pain medication from work. One day while I was at work, a dear friend (Colleen) approached me and asked if I had a problem. I broke down and cried in her arms. I surrendered to her because she created a safe space for me and told me that I wouldn't lose my job if I agreed to go to rehab. I eventually thanked Colleen for saving my life.

Within 3 months I was admitted to a Residential Treatment Center where they had a special program for health professionals. I successfully completed the program and stayed clean for 10 years. However, I ignored the "don't drink" suggestion from my addiction specialist, because I had never craved alcohol before. It wasn't ok. He was right. Eventually, I replaced drugs with alcohol. After rehab it was mandatory to attend weekly follow-up care in a group with other health professionals for 3.5 years. I concurrently attended 12-step meetings, as directed in my return to work contract. I was determined to put this nightmare and all of its complicating issues behind me, instead of accepting my life-long diagnosis. This was evidenced by my not using my real name at meetings. I didn't want anyone to know who I was because I had a professional image to uphold, I thought. I compared myself with the others in the group and determined that my addiction wasn't as bad as theirs. I focused on our differences rather than our similarities. That egotistical decision became detrimental for me. When I returned to work, my contract also required that I tell my coworkers about my addiction. That was extremely hard to do because I was so ashamed. Most of my coworkers were supportive but there were a few that were judgmental. That was enough for me to want this to *all* go away! I relapsed in my 40's. I initiated a 14-week outpatient program, and rejoined the group for addicted health care workers. I attended that weekly for 5 years. I did random urine tests to prove my sobriety because that was one of the conditions to keep my nursing license. My license was initially restricted, and gradually fully restored as a result of my improving recovery.

Throughout the next years of my life, my drinking increased. During this time, I met another man and found myself drinking more. We shared a deep connection; however, our relationship ended abruptly, leaving me feeling destroyed. This was the final straw—the beginning of the end. The rapid downward spiral began. For the next few years I poured alcohol and drugs into my body but nothing cut the pain. I never got counseling for my past trauma because I didn't want to relive it. I couldn't. It didn't take long for others to notice the change in my behavior, as my broken pieces were beginning to show.

Then, to my surprise, my first love (from high school), found me on social media. He was a blessing and I was a hot mess. We had a long-distance relationship, seeing him on weekends, mainly. He would ask me not to drink until he got to my house on a Friday night, but quite often, I couldn't wait. Many times I was inebriated to the point I would be passed out, yet he stayed by my side.

We did not "party" together, I hid it from him as I tried to do with everyone else. All that being said, I absolutely knew that I was an alcoholic/addict. If it wasn't for him, I would have been homeless and destitute. He was asked why he stayed with me and he said, because, I love her with all my heart and if I was ever in the same position, she would stand by me! In life, sometimes the scales are unbalanced, and one person has to bear all the weight in a relationship until balance is restored. He stuck by me, thankfully.

In 2016, I developed a serious and excruciating infection that took 6 months to heal. Due to my history with drugs, my family doctor didn't prescribe adequate pain medication (because he was aware of my addiction). My need for pain medication was denied, so now what? Going to the Emergency room was not an option because I had worked there, (I was shameful) and thought that I would be treated as a drug seeker. My only choice was to look on the streets but I got way more than I was looking for.

Going to a dealer is not like going to a pharmacy; they don't always have what you're looking for. When the pills ran out, I used a variety of illicit drugs in attempt to achieve the same effect. I was reduced to skin and bones and I lost my soul. I had never felt so sick in my life and I knew that if I kept using, I'd die.

My daughter's love and persistence to get me help absolutely saved my life! One day she found a loaded needle in my purse and she knew I was in deadly trouble. Panicked, she gave me an ultimatum. She said, "I will leave you alone if you can look me in the eye and tell me you don't love me," and the addict in me immediately said, "I don't love you." The look in her eyes as she cried and left my room will haunt me for the rest of my life. The thing is, I would have said *anything* to *anyone* in that moment, but she didn't know that. Thankfully, she came back, grabbed the needle, and got rid of it. Later that night, I broke and dislocated my wrist, but don't recall the incident! I didn't know until the next day. Can you imagine that?

The next day my daughters' brought my father to my bedside because they knew that I wouldn't be able to say no if he told me to get help. Bless all of them! My daughter had a bed on standby at "Freedom from Addiction," a private Residential Treatment Center and took out a personal loan in order to have me admitted immediately. When we got there, I vaguely remember a few things during the intake procedure. I was asked to get completely undressed, in front of a female counselor, bend over, and cough to make sure I wasn't smuggling any drugs in my anus or in my vagina. It was humiliating. I have no words.

I spent 10 days in medical detox and then graduated to the 30-day program. This rehab was small, with approximately 15 other clients there at the time, so assistance was available 24/7. Addiction counseling was 1:1 for 8 hours per week. It was intense and difficult but I was able to uncover even more traumatic events that had affected my life. We worked through them one by one.

With my permission, Liz met with my family before I was discharged to make sure that they knew what my new needs would be. She helped me to set up a list of boundaries and helped me to initiate them. I had needed boundaries for decades but never felt that I could implement them.

This rehab also provided "sober coaches." They made a big impact on me because they could relate to me - having walked in my shoes. They helped me work through the big book of Alcoholics Anonymous, accompanied us to 12-step meetings, and provided 1:1 counseling several times per week. Feeling this "brotherhood" was very comforting. For the first time in a long time, I was able to trust someone—that person was Jay Albi. He said what he meant and he meant what he said, making his direction firm and intentional. He was there to help; to give back. He pulled no punches. He was highly respected, and his presence grounded me. It's hard to explain, but he gave me HOPE. Somehow he reminded me of whom I was before drugs and alcohol. I slowly began to crawl out of the hole I was in, as I worked hard to recover.

The rehab also provided alternative therapies such as daily meditation and weekly Reiki treatments to learn how to relax and restore my energy. Relaxation is a crucial part of my recovery because when I'm calm, I can cope by using what I have learned. I know how to stay clean and healthy for myself.

Having to really come to terms with my addiction, I came to recognize things that threaten my recovery. One threat was having access to drugs. It was very difficult to close the door on nursing after having such a long, rewarding career, having drugs within reach was far too tempting. Yes, I could have gotten a different nursing job that didn't have access to drugs, but the memories linger. In my case it was best to close that door. I surrendered my license without regret. My decision was calculated and gave me a sense of relief. Today, I try to help and heal others, just in a different way.

How did I relapse in the past? I severed connections with other people in recovery and didn't reach out when I needed help. I finally stopped trying to get clean and sober by doing it *my way*. My way didn't work.

Why didn't I overdose like my friends did?

Now I'm here for *you*—to help *you* get out of the hole you are in, by jumping in with *you* to help *you* out!

Take addiction seriously, because it won't go away if *you* ignore it.

Please don't have *your* name added to the list of statistics.

> *"The beast in me is sleeping, not dead."*

The anniversary of my clean date is March 14, 2017, and my sober anniversary date is May 5, 2018. I have been nicotine-free since June 11, 2019. I pray that these dates never change.

> *"I choose sober because I wanted a better life.*
> *I stay sober because I got one."*

56. References

(Italics quotes that are not sourced are inspirational things I've heard/learned during my recovery.)

Adlersberg, M., (1997). Chemical dependency: Helping a nurse return to work. *Nursing BC.* (http://www.rnabc.bc.ca/members/nursing-practice/articles/chemical depl.htm). Retrieved May 13, 2021.

Alcohol Withdrawal Syndrome - Wikipedia (2022). (https://en.m.wikipedia.org/wiki/Alcohol_Withdrawal_syndrome). Retrieved March 18, 2022.

Ambivalence - Wikipedia, (2020). (http://www.wikipedia.org). Retrieved January 3rd, 2022).

American Society of Addiction Medicine. (2021). *A Second Chance – An Adventure in Recovery.* (http://www.asam.org). Retrieved July 24, 2021.

American Psychiatric Association (2013). *Diagnostic and Statistical Manual of Mental Disorders,* 5th Edition, pp. 490-491, 2013-2014. (http://www.repository.poltekkes-kaltim.ac.id/657/1/Diagnostic%20and%20statistical%20manual%20of%20mental%20disorders%20_%20DSM-5%%%%20%28%20PDFDrive.com%20%29.pdf. Retrieved March 1, 2022.

Barnwell, B., & Acharya, S. (2014). An integrated understanding of mindfulness, shame, and addiction. Presentation published by Eustace Hutchinson.

Bhasin. H. (2019). How to Be Honest? 14 Ways to Be Honest and Practice Honesty, (http://www.marketing91.com/14-ways-to-be-honest). Retrieved August 15, 2021.

Boogaard, K., (2021). How to Write SMART goals (with examples) – Atlassian. (https://www.atlassian.com/blog/prodctivity/how-to-write-smart-goals/amp). Retrieved March 16, 2022.

Burney, R., (2002), *Inner Child Healing – Why Do It?* (https://codependentrecoveryexpert.wordpress.com/2014/04///28/inner-child-healing-why-do-it/). Retrieved February 20, 2022.

Camp, D., & Lyons, E. (2002), Is low self-esteem an inevitable consequence of stigma? An example from women with chronic mental health problems. *Social Science & Medicine,* 55, 823--834.

Carmona, M. (2022) Alcohol and Anxiety. (https://www.therecoveryvillage.com/mental-health/anxiety-substance-abuse/). *Anxiety & Depression of America, ADAA.* Retrieved March 16, 2022.

Chowdhury, M. (2020), 6 Steps to discover your core values. (https://www.indeed.com/career-advice/career-development/discover-core-values). Retrieved February 20, 2022.

Chui, A. (2021), 53 Relationship questions that will make your love life better. (http://www.lifehack.org). Retrieved October 15, 2021.

Chychula, N., & Sciamanna, C. (2002). Help substance abusers attain and sustain abstinence. *Nurse Practitioner,* 27(11), 30--39. Retrieved May 22, 2021 from ProQuest database.

Craig, H., (2021). 10 ways to build trust in a relationship. (http://www.positivepsychology.com/build-trust). Retrieved November 2, 2021.

Crenshaw, D. A. (1995). 10 Stages of grieving and recovery. *Berevement; Councelling the grieving throughout the life cycle*. Continuum.

Deci, E., & Ryan, R. (2000). Self-determination theory and the facilitation of intrinsic motivation, social development, and well-being. *American Psychologist, 55*(1), 68-78. Retrieved July 14, 2021 from the ProQuest database.

Drake, W. (2021). Guilt Vs. Shame: What's the Difference? (https://www.betterhelp.com). Retrieved November 16, 2021.

Drug Abuse Screening Test, DAST-10, (1982). *The Addiction Research Foundation*. (http://www.bu.edu/bniart/files/2012/04/DAST-10_Institute.pdf Retrieved March 1, 2022.

Drugs, Brains, and Behaviour: The Science of Addiction (2020). National Institute on Drug Abuse. (https://www.drugabuse.gov). Retrieved November 2, 2021.

Gorski, T., (2012). *Post Acute Withdrawal (PAW)*. (http://www.groups..google.com). Retrieved November 5, 2021.

Griffith, J. (1999). Substance abuse disorders in nurses. *Nursing Forum*, 34(4), 19-29. Retrieved November 11, 2021 from ProQuest database.

Hartney, E. (2020). The stages of change model of overcoming addiction. Verywell Mind (http://www.verywellmind.com/the-stages-of-change-model-of-overcoming-addiction-21961). Retrieved November 16, 2021.

International Classification of Diseases, 7th Revision, ICD-7 (1957) (Geneva, Switzerland: World Health Organization).

Lee, A., (2014). 20 Questions to assess your powerlessness & unmanageability, Terminally Forgetful. (http://www.terminallyforgetful.com). Retrieved November 22, 2021.

Maddux, J., & Desmond, D. (2000). Addiction or dependence? *Addiction, 95(5)*, 661--665. Retrieved October 26, 2021 from ProQuest Nursing Journals database.

Maslow's Hierarchy of Needs, (2015). https://goodtherapy.org/Maslows-Hierarchy-of-Needs/Common-therapy-issues). Retrieved March 16, 2022.

Miles, P. (2016). Taking charge of your health & wellbeing. Bakken Center for Spirituality & Healing, University of Minnesota (http://www.takingcharge.csh.umn.edu). Retrieved November 23, 2021.

Moral - Google Dictionary, (2021). Oxford Languages. Retrieved June 8, 2021.

Motivation - Wikipedia, (2021). (http://www.wikipedia.com). Retrieved May 22, 2021.

Nagle, L., (1998). The meaning of technology for people with chronic renal failure. *Holistic Nursing Practice,* 12(4), 78-92. Retrieved July 14, 2021 from the ProQuest database.

Neuroscience of psychoactive substance use and dependence. (2004). World Health Organization. (http://www.scholar.google.ca). Retrieved May 28, 2021.

Pacheco, I. (2018). *The Seven Stages of Grief.* (http://www.recover-from-grief.com). Retrieved May 22, 2021.

Polaris Teen Center, (2018). *Depression and Substance Abuse: Which comes first?* (http://www.polaristeen.com). Retrieved January 3, 2022.

Prochaska, JO & DiClementi, CC. (1986). Toward a comprehensive model of change. In: Treating Addictive Behaviors. *Applied Clinical Psychology. 1986;* 13.

Relapse Symptoms & Behavior - Warning Signs. (2021). (http://www.trihealth.com). Retrieved September 28, 2021.

Prescription Opioids/CAMH, 2022. (https://www.camh.ca/en/health-info/mental-illness-and-addiction-index/prescription-opioids). Retrieved March 12, 2022.

Resentment – Wikipedia. (2021). (http://www.wikipedia.com). Retrieved May 22, 2021.

Salters-Pedneault, K. (2021). Dealing with shame when you have BPD. (https://www.verywellmind.com). Retrieved November 16, 2021.

Signs of Resentment – WebMD. (2020). (http://www.webmd.com-signs-resentment). Retrieved May 22, 2021.

Substance Use and Addiction. Canadian Mental Health Association (2021). (https://www.ontario.cmha.ca/addiction). Retrieved November 28, 2021.

"Understanding Trauma." *Trauma-Informed Practice Guide, pp. 5—7.* Centre of Excellence for Women's Health. (2014). (https://www.bccewh.bc.ca). Retrieved November 17, 2021.

VaderPack. (2020). 10 Spiritual secrets you will learn overtime. (http://www.ifunny.co). Retrieved November 22, 2021.

Villa, L., (2021). Alcohol Prohibition in the U.S. (http://www.recovery.org/alcohol). Retrieved March 11, 2022.

Wesson D. R., & Ling W. (2003), The Clinical Opiate Withdrawal Scale (COWS). *Journal of Psychoactive Drugs,* 35(2), 253—259.

Whalley, M. (2019). *Cognitive Distortions: Unhelpful Thinking Styles.* Psychology Tools. (http://psychologytools.com). Retrieved October 15, 2021.

What Does the Research Say About Reiki? (2016). Bakken Center for Spirituality & Healing, University of Minnesota. (https://takingcharge.csh.umn.edu/explore-healing-practices/reiki/what-does-research-say-about-reiki).

What Is Cognitive Behavioral Therapy? – American Psychological Association, (2017). (http://www.apa.org/ptsd-guideline/patients-and-families/cognitive-behavioral). Retrieved March 15, 2022.

Yerkovich, M., & Yerkovich, K., (2021). *What Is A Love Style?* (http://www.howwelove.com). Retrieved September 6, 2021.

7 Inner Critics, (2019). Barrie and Community. (http://www.barriefht.ca). Retrieved November 15, 2021.

20–Question Addiction Questionnaire John Hopkins, 2017. (http://www.badgeoflifecanada.org/wp-content/uploads/2017/03/20-Questions-Am-I-an-Alcoholic-John-Hopkins.pdf). Retrieved May 22, 2021

www.ingramcontent.com/pod-product-compliance
Lightning Source LLC
Chambersburg PA
CBHW081614100526
44590CB00021B/3436